QUESTIONS AND ANSWERS FOR THE
DIPLOMA IN OCCUPATIONAL MEDICINE

QUESTIONS AND ANSWERS FOR THE

DIPLOMA IN OCCUPATIONAL MEDICINE

SECOND EDITION

CLARE FERNANDES

MBBS, BSc (Hons), DRCOG, DOccMed, MSc (Occupational Medicine), MFOM

Accredited Specialist (Consultant) in Occupational Medicine, Medical Director (EMEA) Haleon Health, Honorary Clinical Lecturer in Occupational Medicine, Manchester University, Co-Founder and Director, The Occupational Health Academy

Scion

© **Scion Publishing Limited, 2025**

Second edition published 2025
Revised edition published 2017
First edition published 2016

All rights, including for text and data mining (TDM), artificial intelligence (AI) training, and similar technologies, are reserved. No part of this book may be reproduced or transmitted, in any form or by any means, without permission.

A CIP catalogue record for this book is available from the British Library.

ISBN 9781914961663

Scion Publishing Limited

The Old Hayloft, Vantage Business Park, Bloxham Road, Banbury OX16 9UX, UK
www.scionpublishing.com

Important Note from the Publisher

The information contained within this book was obtained by Scion Publishing Ltd from sources believed by us to be reliable. However, while every effort has been made to ensure its accuracy, no responsibility for loss or injury whatsoever occasioned to any person acting or refraining from action as a result of information contained herein can be accepted by the authors or publishers.

Readers are reminded that medicine is a constantly evolving science and while the authors and publishers have ensured that all dosages, applications and practices are based on current indications, there may be specific practices which differ between communities. You should always follow the guidelines laid down by the manufacturers of specific products and the relevant authorities in the country in which you are practising.

Although every effort has been made to ensure that all owners of copyright material have been acknowledged in this publication, we would be pleased to acknowledge in subsequent reprints or editions any omissions brought to our attention.

Registered names, trademarks, etc. used in this book, even when not marked as such, are not to be considered unprotected by law.

Typeset by Medlar Publishing Solutions Pvt Ltd, India
Printed in the UK
Last digit is the print number: 10 9 8 7 6 5 4 3 2

Contents

Foreword vii
Preface to the second edition viii
About the author ix
Abbreviations x

Questions for Mock exam 1 .... **1**
   Answers to Mock exam 1 35

Questions for Mock exam 2 .... **95**
   Answers to Mock exam 2 131

Questions for Mock exam 3 .... **189**
   Answers to Mock exam 3 225

Foreword

Preparing for the Diploma in Occupational Medicine requires both a solid understanding of key concepts and the ability to apply them in real-world scenarios. One of the most frequent concerns voiced by delegates on our courses is the limited availability of dedicated exam preparation resources. This second edition of *Questions and Answers for the Diploma in Occupational Medicine* continues to address that need, offering an even more refined and comprehensive approach to revision.

Building on the success of the first edition, this second edition provides an extensive range of questions that reflect the diversity of challenges encountered in both the exam and clinical practice. The inclusion of numerous situational questions is particularly valuable, as these test not only factual knowledge but also the critical thinking and decision-making skills essential for occupational health professionals. The book's structured mock exam format simulates the actual Diploma assessment, allowing candidates to familiarise themselves with the style and rigour of the exam while developing their confidence under realistic conditions.

Beyond the exam, occupational medicine plays a crucial role in safeguarding the health and wellbeing of workers. As the specialty evolves, the demand for skilled professionals continues to grow, making the contributions of future diplomats all the more vital. This book not only aids in exam success but also serves as a stepping stone into a dynamic and rewarding career.

Whether used for independent study or as a supplement to formal training, this book remains an essential resource for building knowledge, refining understanding, and shaping the next generation of occupational health professionals.

Dr Lanre Ogunyemi
FRCSEd FACOEM FFOMI FFOM FRCPI FRCP

Consultant in Occupational Medicine
President, Society of Occupational Medicine, UK
Academic Registrar (Chief Examiner),
Faculty of Occupational Medicine of the RCP Ireland
Medical Director & Course Lead, TOPHS Ltd

Preface to the second edition

The first edition of this book was born from necessity being the mother of invention. In 2014, preparing for the Diploma in Occupational Medicine and faced with a scarcity of revision materials, I developed a personal study aid. What began as a private resource evolved into a best-selling revision guide. I am honoured that the *Journal of Occupational Medicine* (April 2018) recognised the first edition as "an excellent investment for anyone preparing for the exam", and it has been humbling to learn that the book has been used as far afield as Malaysia, India and New Zealand.

This second edition expands upon its predecessor, incorporating important updates to legislation and guidance, while integrating valuable feedback from readers who used the book for examination preparation. I have enriched the content with authentic clinical scenarios that colleagues and I have encountered, concentrating on prevalent and significant contemporary Occupational Health concerns.

This edition has been organised into three mock examinations, enabling candidates to practise under timed conditions simulating the actual examination, should they choose. Throughout, I have included references to key resources that supplement revision effectively, emphasising predominantly free materials that will be beneficial to candidates. Where possible, each question deliberately asks for the "most appropriate" or "most correct" answer to more accurately mimic the exam; answers are accompanied by comprehensive explanations of why the designated answer represents the optimal choice. My main objective remains consistent – to provide a clear, structured resource supporting those pursuing careers in Occupational Health.

Answers to questions in the book were checked for accuracy by Dr Sam Goodall. Dr Goodall is an ST5 in Occupational Medicine and an honorary clinical lecturer in Occupational Health at the University of Manchester, and works in an NHS occupational health department. I would like to extend my thanks to Dr Goodall for verifying the currency and accuracy of the clinical guidelines.

To my mentors and colleagues: thank you for your support and company on my Occupational Health journey.

Good luck, and welcome to Occupational Medicine.

Clare Fernandes

About the author

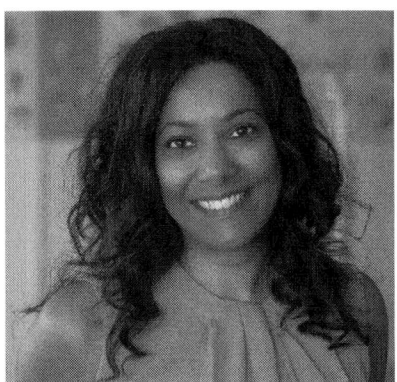

Dr Clare Fernandes combines her expertise as an accredited specialist in Occupational Medicine with her extensive international experience across diverse industries, including pivotal roles at the BBC and Haleon. With a passion for teaching and having achieved a distinction in her MSc in Occupational Medicine, she serves as an honorary lecturer in Occupational Medicine at Manchester University. As the co-founder of the Occupational Health Academy, she developed the premier revision course for the Diploma in Occupational Medicine. Her book encapsulates this wealth of knowledge and experience, making it an indispensable resource for Diploma candidates.

Abbreviations

Acas	The Advisory, Conciliation and Arbitration Service
APF	assigned protection factor
BBV	blood-borne virus
BCC	basal cell carcinoma
BMGV	biological monitoring guidance value
BMI	body mass index
CI	confidence interval
COPD	chronic obstructive pulmonary disease
COSHH	Control of Substances Hazardous to Health
CTS	carpal tunnel syndrome
DD	Dupuytren's disease
DSE	display screen equipment
DVLA	Driver and Vehicle Licensing Agency
EAV	exposure action value
EFAW	Emergency First Aid at Work
ELV	exposure limit value
EMAS	Employment Medical Advisory Service
ENT	ear, nose and throat
EPP	exposure-prone procedure
EqA	Equality Act
ET	employment tribunal
FAW	First Aid at Work
FEV_1	forced expiratory volume in 1 second
FN	false negative
FOM	Faculty of Occupational Medicine
FVC	forced vital capacity
GDPR	General Data Protection Regulations
GMC	General Medical Council
GP	general practitioner
HASAWA	Health and Safety at Work etc. Act (1974)
HAVS	hand arm vibration syndrome
HBV	hepatitis B virus
HCV	hepatitis C virus
HCW	healthcare worker
HIV	human immunodeficiency virus
HP	hypersensitivity pneumonitis
HR	Human Resources

HSE	Health and Safety Executive
IARC	International Agency for Research on Cancer
IIAC	Industrial Injuries Advisory Council
IIDB	Industrial Injuries Disablement Benefit
IR	ionising radiation
IVF	*in vitro* fertilisation
MS	multiple sclerosis
MSD	musculoskeletal disorders
ND	neurodifferent
NHS	National Health Service
OA	occupational asthma
OAE	otoacoustic emission
OH	occupational health
OHP	occupational health physician
PD	prescribed disease
PEF	peak expiratory flow
PPE	personal protective equipment
PPV	positive predictive value
PVC	polyvinyl chloride
RCS	respirable crystalline silica
RCT	randomised controlled trial
RIDDOR	Reporting of Injuries, Diseases and Dangerous Occurrences Regulations
RPE	respiratory protection equipment
RR	relative risk
RTW	return to work
SAR	Subject Access Request
SBS	sick building syndrome
SEQOHS	Safe, Effective, Quality Occupational Health Service
STEL	short-term exposure limit
TB	tuberculosis
TIA	transient ischaemic attack
TP	true positive
TTS	temporary threshold shift
TWA	time-weighted average
UV	ultraviolet
VCM	vinyl chloride monomer
VZV	varicella zoster virus
WBV	whole body vibration
WEL	workplace exposure limit

QUESTIONS for Mock exam 1

QUESTION 1

You take a group of occupational health (OH) trainees on a workplace visit to a workshop where paint spraying with isocyanate-containing paint is used. One worker shows you his test results which say that 'di-amines are not present in his urine'.

A student asks you what type of test this is. What is the most appropriate answer?

a) Biological effect monitoring
b) Biological monitoring
c) A drug test
d) Health screening
e) Health surveillance

QUESTION 2

You are assessing an employee who has developed skin lesions after prolonged dioxin exposure. On examination, there are open comedones on the cheeks.

Which of the following is the most likely diagnosis?

a) Allergic contact dermatitis
b) Psoriasis
c) Acne vulgaris
d) Chloracne
e) Seborrhoeic dermatitis

QUESTION 3

A construction worker who recently had surgery for Dupuytren's disease is preparing to return to work. He is concerned about the possibility of his symptoms recurring due to his exposure to vibrating tools.

What is the most appropriate advice for him regarding his return to work?

a) Recurrence of symptoms is more likely after returning to work with vibrating tools, so he should avoid such tasks
b) There is no existing evidence indicating that using vibrating tools at work raises the risk of symptoms returning
c) He should delay returning to work until more research on the effects of vibrating tools is available
d) Recurrence of symptoms is guaranteed if he resumes tasks involving vibration
e) He should be redeployed to a different role to avoid tasks involving vibrating tools

QUESTION 4

You are the occupational health (OH) practitioner for an ambulance service. A staff member was exposed to both hepatitis B and hepatitis C in the line of duty and has attended your clinic for post-exposure counselling. She asks when her first test for hepatitis B and C will be.

What is the most appropriate response?

a) Immediately after exposure
b) 1 week after exposure
c) 6 weeks after exposure
d) 3 months after exposure
e) 1 year after exposure

QUESTION 5

You are working with a renovation firm reviewing the requirements for maintaining the asbestos health records for their operatives. The Human Resources department is unclear about how long these records need to be kept for.

For how long must asbestos health records be kept?

a) 10 years
b) 20 years
c) 30 years
d) 40 years
e) Until the employee's 75th birthday

QUESTION 6

You are a medical educator teaching a class about occupational health. During the lecture, you present a case study about a 58-year-old male who has been diagnosed with lung cancer after working for 30 years in an environment with heavy asbestos exposure. The class discusses various carcinogens and their International Agency for Research on Cancer (IARC) classifications.

Which IARC classification indicates that an agent is known to be carcinogenic to humans?

a) Group 1
b) Group 2A
c) Group 2B
d) Group 3
e) Group 4

QUESTION 7

A 45-year-old employee is seeking reasonable adjustments at work due to a chronic condition. The employee has not received a formal medical diagnosis but reports significant limitations in daily activities due to pain and fatigue. The employer is unsure whether the employee qualifies for reasonable adjustments under the law, given the lack of a specific diagnosis.

When determining whether this employee qualifies for reasonable adjustments under disability legislation, which of the following is most relevant to consider?

a) The presence of a formal diagnosis
b) Whether the impairment is physical or mental
c) Employee compliance with investigations and/or treatment
d) The effect of the impairment
e) The type of symptoms experienced

QUESTION 8

You are an occupational physician assessing a 55-year-old factory worker who has severe chronic obstructive pulmonary disease (COPD). Despite his condition, he believes he can continue his physically demanding job without any changes or restrictions. You are concerned that his severe COPD significantly limits his ability to safely perform his duties and believe that he should be redeployed to a sedentary role. During the assessment, the worker strongly expresses his desire to remain in his current role without modifications and resists any suggestion of changing his job responsibilities.

What is the most appropriate action to take?

a) Opine that he is fit for work without adjustments, respecting his wishes
b) Recommend medical retirement as a compromise
c) Document the worker's views but explain your opinion that redeployment is needed
d) Ignore the worker's preferences and speak to the manager about redeploying him to a different role
e) Allow the worker to dictate his job placement decision, as his autonomy should be prioritised

QUESTION 9

You are running a careers session for doctors interested in occupational medicine. During the session, a doctor asks about the requirements for conducting medical examinations for seafarers.

Which one of the following types of doctor are authorised to carry out seafarer medical examinations?

a) Maritime and Coastguard Agency (MCA) Approved Doctors
b) Health and Safety Executive (HSE) Appointed Doctors
c) Any doctor with the Diploma in Occupational Medicine qualification
d) Any Accredited Specialist in occupational medicine
e) Any General Practitioner

QUESTION 10

You are assisting an employer in reviewing their guidance on procedures for noise health surveillance. The current guidance advises employees to wait 10 hours after exposure to loud noise before undergoing surveillance audiometry. However, you identify that this recommendation does not align with best practice, which aims to minimise the influence of temporary threshold shifts (TTS) on audiometry results.

How should the guidance be amended to align with best practice for noise health surveillance?

a) Change the waiting period to 8 hours after noise exposure
b) Maintain the waiting period at 10 hours after noise exposure
c) Change the waiting period to 14 hours after noise exposure
d) Change the waiting period to 16 hours after noise exposure
e) Change the waiting period to 24 hours after noise exposure

QUESTION 11

You are reviewing the occupational health risks associated with welding.

Which one of the following infections are welders at an increased risk of developing due to their occupation?

a) Hepatitis B virus
b) *Mycobacterium tuberculosis*
c) *Streptococcus pneumoniae*
d) *Legionella pneumophila*
e) SARS-CoV-2

QUESTION 12

You are reviewing a case involving a 38-year-old welder who reports a sudden onset of eye pain, tearing, and redness after working on a welding project. The worker describes the sensation as feeling like he has "sand in the eye" and mentions a high sensitivity to light.

What is the most likely cause of this worker's symptoms?

a) Chemical exposure
b) Ultraviolet (UV) radiation

c) Dust particles
d) Infrared radiation
e) Bacterial infection

QUESTION 13

A 55-year-old woman presents with numbness, tingling and pain in her hands, which worsens at night. On examination, you suspect carpal tunnel syndrome (CTS).

Which one of the following is a constitutional risk factor for developing carpal tunnel syndrome?

a) Diabetes
b) Low body mass index (BMI)
c) Alcohol use
d) Poor hand hygiene
e) Sedentary lifestyle

QUESTION 14

A 45-year-old office worker was scheduled for health surveillance required by their employer. However, the employee did not attend the scheduled appointment. As an independent practitioner, you are considering whether to inform the employer about the missed appointment.

Which one of the following statements is true regarding informing an employer about an employee's failure to attend an appointment?

a) You must obtain the employee's consent before informing the employer about the missed appointment
b) Informing the employer about the missed health assessment does not require the employee's consent
c) You should only inform the employer about the missed appointment if the employee has given prior consent
d) Informing the employer of the missed appointment can only be done if you have a legal obligation to do so
e) The employee's consent is required to inform the employer, but you may proceed without it if you believe it is in the public interest

QUESTION 15

You are an OH professional advising a healthcare worker (HCW) on the categorisation of their clinical procedures to assess the risk of exposure-prone procedures (EPPs).

Which one of the following is classified as a Category 3 EPP?

a) Local anaesthetic injection in dentistry
b) Routine tooth extraction
c) Hysterectomy
d) Rigid sigmoidoscopy including biopsy
e) Removal of haemorrhoids

QUESTION 16

You are shadowing at an occupational lung disease clinic. A 50-year-old engineer in the aerospace industry presents with shortness of breath, unexplained coughing, fatigue, weight loss, fever and night sweats. Imaging reveals florid non-caseating granulomatous lung disease.

What is the most likely occupational exposure that would cause his symptoms?

a) Beryllium
b) Cadmium
c) Cobalt
d) *Mycobacterium tuberculosis*
e) Silica

QUESTION 17

An aviary has become aware of a psittacosis outbreak at the local zoo, including an infection in staff. They contact you to help them avoid this affecting their business.

Using the hierarchy of control, which of the following actions is the most effective way to reduce the risk of an outbreak?

a) Ensure good ventilation in bird housing
b) Good occupational hygiene practices should be followed, particularly washing hands with soap and warm water

c) Isolate sick birds from the rest of the flock
d) Regularly clean bird cages with high-pressure jet washing
e) Wear suitable protective clothing when handling birds or cleaning cages

QUESTION 18

You are advising a local council that has identified high rates of work-related stress, reducing their employee retention rates. As part of their plan to reduce employee ill health, they have updated their bullying and harassment policy.

Which one of the Health and Safety Executive (HSE) Management Standards does this action address?

a) Control
b) Demands
c) Relationships
d) Role
e) Support

QUESTION 19

You encounter a 35-year-old baker presenting with symptoms suggestive of occupational asthma.

Which investigation should be pursued next to establish a diagnosis?

a) Chest X-ray
b) Inhalation challenge
c) Serial peak flows
d) Spirometry
e) Workplace challenge

QUESTION 20

You are an OH doctor for a local charity. An employee who has a diagnosis of secondary progressive multiple sclerosis (MS) and now needs to use a wheelchair, requests that a lift be installed so she can access the upper floors of the workplace where she works. After conducting a cost-analysis exercise, the employer finds that installing a lift would be unaffordable for the business. The employer seeks your advice on how to proceed in compliance with the Equality Act 2010.

What is the most appropriate advice to give the employer?

a) Suggest the employee work from home permanently as a reasonable adjustment
b) Suggest that the employee's request is denied but explore modifying her role so she can work on the ground floor
c) Suggest that the employee's request needs to be enacted as she falls under the disability provisions of the Equality Act
d) Suggest that the employee applies to the Access to Work Scheme for funding the building of a lift
e) Suggest that the employee's request is unreasonable and redeploy her to a role that does not require access to upper floors

QUESTION 21

You are evaluating a 60-year-old gardener who has been referred for consideration of ill-health retirement due to long Covid. During the examination, you notice a 2 cm lesion on his face with a rolled, pearly edge and central ulceration.

What is the most likely occupational exposure that could cause this type of lesion?

a) Anthrax
b) Tinea
c) Ultraviolet (UV) radiation
d) Latex
e) Celery

QUESTION 22

You are speaking to a group of trainee occupational physicians about the long-term effects of chemical exposures, focusing on vinyl chloride monomer (VCM), a substance used in the production of polyvinyl chloride (PVC).

Which of the following is a long-term health effect associated with chronic exposure to VCM?

a) Hepatocellular carcinoma
b) Angiosarcoma of the liver
c) Acro-osteolysis

d) Non-cirrhotic portal fibrosis
e) All of the above

QUESTION 23

A 43-year-old care worker comes to you with a one-year history of fibromyalgia. She has found it increasingly difficult to concentrate due to 'brain fog' and continues to find shift work difficult because of fatigue. She has not seen occupational health previously, and no action has been taken at work to date. She wishes to be considered for ill-health retirement.

Which one of the following is the most appropriate next step to be considered in her management?

a) Adjustments
b) Ill-health retirement
c) Redeployment
d) Refer to a senior colleague
e) Sick leave until symptom resolution

QUESTION 24

You see an employee in clinic who works with 3D printers. He tells you that he thinks working with this machine has caused his diagnosis of psoriasis.

In evaluating whether an occupational exposure is linked to a particular disease, you are considering the Bradford Hill criteria.

Which of the following best describes the use of the criterion 'Analogy'?

a) Assessing whether the exposure precedes the onset of the disease
b) Determining if similar exposures are known to cause the disease in other settings or populations
c) Examining if there is a dose–response relationship between the exposure and the disease
d) Checking if the association between exposure and disease is consistent across different studies
e) Whether the exposure is associated with a specific disease and not with other unrelated diseases

QUESTION 25

Mr Smith is a manager working in the nuclear industry where many workers are industrial radiographers. Mr Smith is concerned about the potential health risks associated with radiation exposure and wants to ensure that all staff are correctly designated as classified workers where appropriate.

Under the Ionising Radiations Regulations 2017, which one of the following is true regarding the designation of classified workers?

a) It is up to the employee to decide if they are a classified worker
b) It is the duty of the employer to designate an individual as a classified worker
c) It is the occupational health doctor's responsibility to classify workers
d) Classified worker status is automatically assigned to anyone exposed to ionising radiation
e) The Health and Safety Executive (HSE) is responsible for classifying workers

QUESTION 26

An employer is evaluating dust exposure in the workplace and needs to understand the term 'inhalable dust' to better assess potential health risks.

Which one of the following is the definition of 'inhalable dust'?

a) Dust particles that are small enough to reach the lungs and cause damage to the respiratory system
b) Dust that can enter the nose and mouth during breathing, including particles that may cause damage to the upper respiratory tract
c) Dust particles that may cause damage to the upper respiratory tract
d) Dust particles that are too large to be inhaled and therefore do not pose a risk to respiratory health
e) Total dust levels in the workplace

QUESTION 27

You are the lead physician responsible for an OH service at a large manufacturing company. The company deals with hazardous materials and heavy machinery. During a recent safety audit, you identified several gaps in the company's first aid provisions, including inadequate first aid kits and a lack of trained first aid personnel.

Which would be the best action to take next?

a) Directly implement first aid training and purchase the necessary first aid supplies
b) Advise the employer on the specific first aid requirements and the need to address the identified gaps
c) Report the company to the Health and Safety Executive (HSE) for failing to meet first aid standards
d) Arrange for external first aid providers to take over the company's first aid responsibilities
e) Take no action, as the duty of providing first aid lies solely with the employer

QUESTION 28

An employer at a brewery has conducted a risk assessment before commencing work, which has identified the need for health surveillance. As part of establishing a health surveillance programme, the employer asks you about the primary purpose of health surveillance.

What is the most appropriate answer?

a) To provide feedback on the accuracy of the risk assessment
b) To act as part of the employer's control measures
c) To check effectiveness of control measures
d) To diagnose work-related ill health
e) To detect adverse health effects at an early stage

QUESTION 29

You are an OH professional conducting a workplace assessment for a large corporate office. Part of your evaluation includes ensuring that the lighting in the office is adequate for the tasks performed by the staff, which mostly involve computer work and reading documents.

What is the recommended average illuminance (lux) level for an office environment to ensure safe and effective work performance?

a) 1–200 lux
b) 200–500 lux
c) 500–1000 lux
d) 1000–1500 lux
e) Over 1500 lux

QUESTION 30

A construction worker has been using a vibrating hand tool for the past five years. Recently, he has started experiencing symptoms such as numbness and tingling in his fingers. During your assessment, you review the workplace safety guidelines and vibration exposure levels.

What is generally accepted to be the 'no harm level' of exposure when working with vibrating handheld tools?

a) 0.5 m/sec^2
b) 1 m/sec^2
c) 2.5 m/sec^2
d) 3.0 m/sec^2
e) 4.0 m/sec^2

QUESTION 31

A pregnant worker in an organisation has been exposed to a risk that could potentially harm her or her unborn child. After assessing the situation, the employer finds that they are unable to control or remove the risk.

What should be the best next steps to ensure the worker's health and safety?

a) Immediately suspend the worker without pay
b) Offer suitable alternative work that is appropriate for the pregnant worker on the same terms and conditions
c) Continue with the current working conditions and monitor the situation, providing no additional adjustments
d) Adjust the working conditions or hours to avoid the risk
e) Suspend the worker on paid leave

QUESTION 32

You are reviewing the occupational health risks associated with sewage exposure.

Which of the following infections are sewage workers at an increased risk of developing due to their occupation?

a) Hepatitis A virus
b) Hepatitis B virus

c) Hepatitis C virus
d) Hepatitis D virus
e) Hepatitis E virus

QUESTION 33

A company is seeking information on national trends in work-related ill health to better understand the risks in their industry. They are directed to a surveillance scheme specifically designed to monitor the incidence of work-related health conditions in the UK.

Which of the following surveillance schemes has the primary aim of monitoring the incidence and trends in work-related ill health?

a) The Labour Force Survey (LFS)
b) The Health and Occupation Research (THOR) network
c) The Workplace Employment Relations Study (WERS)
d) The European Working Conditions Survey (EWCS)
e) The National Health Service (NHS) Patient Safety Alert System

QUESTION 34

You see a 29-year-old welder who has been referred for frequent, short sickness absences. On further enquiry she describes fever, shivering and headache, and malaise that she feels occurs in the evening after she is at work. She has not needed any treatment for these symptoms, which she has attributed to viral illness. She has no other past medical history.

What is the most likely diagnosis?

a) COPD
b) Influenza
c) Metal fume fever
d) Occupational asthma
e) Welder's lung

QUESTION 35

You have been asked to see a 52-year-old personal assistant with sporadic wheezy episodes whilst at work.

What is the next practical step you should take?

a) Speak to his managers about his work environment
b) Take a detailed history
c) Inspect his workplace
d) Request his previous medical history from his general practitioner
e) Request a chest X-ray

QUESTION 36

Researchers are interested in understanding the relationship between past occupational exposure and the development of a disease with a long latency period.

Which type of study design is most appropriate for investigating this?

a) Cross-sectional study
b) Ecological study
c) Case–control study
d) Prospective cohort study
e) Randomised controlled trial

QUESTION 37

You meet with unions at a construction company. They want to talk to you about the health effects of diesel exhaust fumes, to which they feel they are heavily exposed. They are particularly concerned about the risk of cancer.

What is the cancer most associated with diesel fumes?

a) Bladder
b) Bowel
c) Lung
d) Ovarian
e) Prostate

QUESTION 38

You are conducting an OH assessment for a 20-year-old employee recently diagnosed with relapsing–remitting multiple sclerosis (MS) who has experienced complete remission since diagnosis.

What is the most appropriate advice to provide regarding the Equality Act?

a) She is not covered by the Equality Act because she currently does not have symptoms
b) She is covered by the Equality Act only after being employed for at least 2 years
c) She is covered by the Equality Act immediately upon her diagnosis
d) The Equality Act applies only if her MS symptoms reoccur in the future
e) The Equality Act applies only if she requires reasonable adjustments at work

QUESTION 39

You see a 56-year-old tree surgeon who has been referred with numbness and tingling in both hands and episodic blanching of his fingers associated with cold weather. You take a history and examine him, and take his blood pressure. You examine his grip strength and check sensation of his fingers.

What is the next test that is most appropriate?

a) Finger systolic blood pressure test
b) Finger rewarming after cold provocation
c) Purdue peg board
d) Nerve conduction study
e) Doppler ultrasound

QUESTION 40

Which one of the following entities is primarily responsible for enforcing health and safety law in the UK?

a) The Department for Work and Pensions (DWP)
b) The Health and Safety Executive (HSE)
c) The Environment Agency (EA)
d) The Employment Tribunals (ET)
e) The National Health Service (NHS)

QUESTION 41

You are collaborating with the safety team to evaluate the outcomes of a recent manual handling risk assessment for a group of warehouse workers. A system of manual handling aids has been introduced to facilitate easier transportation of boxes.

What is the most appropriate next step under manual handling regulations as part of the risk assessment process?

a) Instigate a statutory health surveillance programme
b) No further action needed
c) Review any ongoing sickness absence due to musculoskeletal disease
d) Review the risk assessment in one year
e) Undertake individual risk assessments

QUESTION 42

A 30-year-old laboratory technician has been exposed to a chemical spill in the lab. The spill was quickly contained, but the technician was exposed to a low concentration of the chemical for an extended period before the area was ventilated. You are reviewing the incident to determine the potential health impact of the exposure.

Which of the following best explains how the total dose of chemical exposure is calculated in this scenario?

a) Dose = Concentration ÷ Time
b) Dose = Concentration × Time
c) Dose = Concentration + Time
d) Dose = Time ÷ Concentration
e) Dose = Concentration − Time

QUESTION 43

You see Mr Jones, a postal worker who was referred for advice regarding his return to work. Mr Jones tells you that he went off sick after he was bitten by a dog while delivering a parcel. He required antibiotics and stitches but was not admitted to hospital. He has been absent for two weeks to date. His wound is healing well.

Which of the following is the most appropriate advice for you to give the employer regarding the Reporting of Injuries, Diseases and Dangerous Occurrences Regulations 2013 (RIDDOR)?

a) This incident is not RIDDOR reportable
b) This is RIDDOR reportable as a dangerous occurrence
c) This is RIDDOR reportable as he has had more than 7 days of absence due to the incident
d) You should not provide advice on RIDDOR as this is not an occupational health disease
e) You should not provide advice on RIDDOR as you are not responsible for reporting these to the HSE

QUESTION 44

You are seeing a 34-year-old park ranger to give advice on his return to work. He describes sickness absence due to flu-like illness with a "bull's-eye" rash, which needed treatment with antibiotics.

What is the most likely diagnosis?

a) Cellulitis
b) Erythema multiforme
c) Lyme disease
d) Orf
e) Ringworm

QUESTION 45

You receive a query from a new administrator in your occupational health company. She has received a call from a client where you undertake health surveillance for vibration exposure. The administrator informs you that one of the employees has completed their annual questionnaire which indicates that they need further assessment.

Which tier of surveillance for hand arm vibration syndrome (HAVS) is the most appropriate next step?

a) Tier 1
b) Tier 2
c) Tier 3

d) Tier 4
e) Tier 5

QUESTION 46

You see a 25-year-old abattoir worker who has been referred by management for advice following his recent diagnosis of attention deficit hyperactivity disorder (ADHD). You notice a lesion on his hand, which he explained started as an "insect bite" and then became a blister. On examination, there is a 3 cm ulcer surrounded by small blisters with marked swelling of the surrounding skin with a central black scab.

What is the most likely diagnosis?

a) Anthrax
b) Lyme disease
c) Insect bite
d) Malignant melanoma
e) Orf

QUESTION 47

You are the occupational health physician (OHP) conducting a health promotion session at a battery production facility. During the session, an employee asks about the link between cadmium exposure and cancer.

Which of the following cancers is associated with cadmium exposure?

a) Lung
b) Prostate
c) Pancreas
d) Renal
e) All of the above

QUESTION 48

A 30-year-old female laboratory technician presents to the occupational health clinic with concerns about various hazards in her workplace. She works with chemicals and biological samples, and occasionally handles radiation equipment. Recently, she experienced a minor chemical spill, which led her to reflect on the different hazards she faces daily and their potential risks.

Which one of the following best describes the different categories of hazards she might encounter in her workplace?

a) Biological, chemical, ergonomic, physical and psychosocial hazards
b) Biological, chemical, environmental, genetic and psychosocial hazards
c) Chemical, ergonomic, genetic, physical and psychosocial hazards
d) Biological, environmental, ergonomic, physical and psychosocial hazards
e) Chemical, environmental, genetic, physical and psychosocial hazards

QUESTION 49

You are being shadowed by a medical student. You see a 60-year-old truck driver with a recent diagnosis of epilepsy is undergoing a fitness to drive medical by the occupational health team. The student wants to understand the regulations set by the Driver and Vehicle Licensing Agency (DVLA) regarding the risk of sudden disabling events.

According to DVLA guidelines, what is the maximum acceptable risk of a sudden disabling event in one year in this driver?

a) 20% likelihood of an event
b) 10% likelihood of an event
c) 5% likelihood of an event
d) 2% likelihood of an event
e) 1% likelihood of an event

QUESTION 50

You are advising a 36-year-old employee who is pregnant with twins and has had an uncomplicated pregnancy. She wishes to take a 2-hour flight to attend a work-related conference. She will be 22 weeks pregnant. Her employer is seeking guidance on whether she should go.

Considering the general advice for twin pregnancies, what is the most appropriate recommendation?

a) The employee can undertake the flight as planned, as there are no specific restrictions for twin pregnancies at 22 weeks
b) The employee should be advised not to fly, as twin pregnancies are generally advised to avoid flying after 22 weeks

c) The employee can undertake the flight, but she should consult her healthcare provider for personalised advice
d) The employee should be advised to reschedule the conference to avoid any potential risks associated with flying during pregnancy
e) The employee should seek advice from her airline about their policies on flying with a twin pregnancy, as policies might vary

QUESTION 51

You are the OHP for a local foundry. You have seen a significant increase in workers experiencing heat stress due to high ambient temperatures and thermal radiation in their workplace. Management seeks the best option to mitigate these health risks. They have provided several solutions that they can feasibly implement.

What is the most appropriate way to reduce the risk of heat stress in these workers?

a) Acclimatising employees
b) Improving air movement
c) Incorporating rest periods
d) Providing a water cooler
e) Protective clothing

QUESTION 52

You are undertaking a workplace visit at a workplace involving welding. One of your students notices a sign on the local exhaust ventilation which states that the last inspection was 12 months ago. The manager assures you that the equipment is in a good state of repair.

When should the business schedule the next inspection?

a) 2 months
b) 6 months
c) 12 months
d) 2 years
e) 4 years

QUESTION 53

You advise a company on their health surveillance for noise. An employee is moving into a role located within a hearing protection zone. The company wants to know when he should commence participation in the health surveillance programme.

What is the most appropriate response?

a) He does not need health surveillance
b) He should have started in the health surveillance programme when he started work with the company
c) He needs to have a health surveillance review annually for the first 2 years of employment
d) In 3 years
e) It is appropriate to have a health surveillance review prior to starting in the new job role

QUESTION 54

You are asked to give an opinion on fitness to work for a veterinary surgeon who is 15 weeks pregnant. It is birthing season at the farm where she works. She is worried about exposure to *Coxiella burnetii*.

What is the most appropriate opinion to give?

a) She is fit to work with no adjustments
b) She needs to be removed from delivering calves and lambs
c) She needs to be removed from delivering lambs
d) She needs to be removed from delivering calves
e) She needs to be redeployed from all work with animals

QUESTION 55

You are an OH professional evaluating an office environment where several employees have reported symptoms such as headaches, dizziness and eye irritation. Some of the staff believe these symptoms are caused by the building environment, and there is concern that this might indicate a serious workplace illness.

Which of the following statements best describes 'sick building syndrome'?

a) Sick building syndrome is a recognised medical condition that can be precisely diagnosed
b) Sick building syndrome should be diagnosed in workplaces where there are clusters of cases of specific illnesses like legionnaires' disease and humidifier fever
c) Sick building syndrome refers to a set of symptoms reported by building occupants that cannot be traced to a specific illness or hazard
d) Sick building syndrome is caused by long-term exposure to cumulative hazards such as asbestos and radon
e) Sick building syndrome is a condition caused by adverse physical conditions such as excessive noise, heat or cold

QUESTION 56

You see a 52-year-old office worker who has been referred one week after a transient ischaemic attack (TIA) for advice on return to work. He is eager to return to his routine, and commutes for one hour each day by car for employment.

What is the most appropriate advice regarding his return to driving?

a) He can resume driving immediately since he has had no further episodes
b) He must not drive for 1 month after a TIA and does not need to notify the DVLA
c) He must not drive for 3 months after a TIA and must notify the DVLA
d) He must not drive for 6 months after a TIA and must notify the DVLA
e) He must not drive for 1 year after a TIA and must notify the DVLA

QUESTION 57

A 50-year-old employee has recently been evaluated by you for a work-related health issue, and a report has been prepared for their employer stating that the employee is fit for work. The patient now wishes to withdraw consent for the report to be disclosed to their employer, expressing disagreement with your opinion that they are fit to work.

What is the most appropriate course of action if an employee withdraws consent for the disclosure of a report?

a) Disclose the report to the employer anyway, as the report has been paid for and may be important for the employer
b) Notify the report commissioner of the employee's withdrawal of consent, but withhold the report and do not disclose any further information
c) Amend the report to reflect the employee's disagreement and disclose it to the employer
d) Inform the employee that their withdrawal of consent will not be honoured and disclose the report to the employer as planned
e) Disclose the report to the employer without the employee's consent, citing that it contains factual information regarding their fitness for work

QUESTION 58

You are working with the safety team, evaluating a risk assessment of a workplace using toluene.

The workers are using respiratory protection equipment (RPE) with an assigned protection factor (APF) of 200.

The measured airborne toluene concentration: 500 ppm (parts per million) within an 8-hour time-weighted average (TWA).

Toluene WEL (workplace exposure limit): 50 ppm (from EH40).

What is the lowest assigned protection factor that should be used for the employee's respiratory protection equipment?

a) 4
b) 10
c) 20
d) 40
e) 2000

QUESTION 59

You are the OHP reviewing the health questionnaire of a pregnant nurse prior to starting work on the renal ward. She has no history of chickenpox or shingles, nor vaccination/passive immunity against VZV.

What is the most appropriate next step in managing this pregnant healthcare worker's potential exposure to VZV (varicella zoster virus)?

a) Advise her to avoid patient contact until after her pregnancy
b) Clear her to work without restrictions
c) Offer VZV immunoglobulin (VZIG)
d) Test her for VZV antibodies
e) No further action is required as there is no history of chickenpox or shingles

QUESTION 60

A health and safety officer is conducting a health promotion seminar for office workers who use display screen equipment (DSE). During the seminar, one of the employees asks about the most common health problems associated with DSE work.

Which of the following health problems is related to DSE work?

a) Epilepsy
b) Miscarriage
c) Permanent eye damage
d) Upper limb disorders
e) All of the above

QUESTION 61

You are working as a contractor at a car manufacturing site. The employer wants you to help assess the ergonomic risks on the assembly line.

What is the most appropriate tool to use?

a) ART tool
b) RAPP tool
c) MAC tool
d) QRISK tool
e) V-MAC tool

QUESTION 62

A 45-year-old male construction worker visits the clinic for health surveillance. During the examination, he expresses concerns about his workplace, specifically about the potential for asbestos exposure. He has read that asbestos is dangerous and is worried about the implications for his health.

What is the most appropriate way to explain the difference between hazard and risk in the context of his concern about asbestos exposure?

a) Hazard refers to the inherent potential of asbestos to cause harm, whereas risk is the likelihood that this harm will occur given the level of exposure
b) Hazard is the actual health effect experienced by the worker, while risk is the hypothetical probability of experiencing this effect
c) Hazard involves the environmental presence of asbestos, and risk is related to the individual's genetic predisposition to asbestos-related diseases
d) Hazard describes the severity of the potential health effects, while risk refers to the measures taken to prevent exposure
e) Hazard and risk are interchangeable terms used to describe the potential for asbestos to cause health problems

QUESTION 63

You are an OHP assessing a 60-year-old ex-construction worker who has recently been diagnosed with lung cancer, believed to be related to prolonged asbestos exposure. The worker is seeking advice on their eligibility for the Industrial Injuries Disablement Benefit (IIDB) and wants to understand the criteria for receiving this benefit.

To qualify for the IIDB, what is the minimum level of disability (expressed as a percentage) that this worker needs to be assessed as having?

a) All workers with a prescribed disease in the appropriate occupation are entitled to benefits regardless of the level of disability
b) The worker must be assessed as at least 14% disabled
c) The worker must be assessed as at least 25% disabled
d) The worker must be assessed as at least 50% disabled
e) The worker must have a total loss of work capability, regardless of the percentage of disability

QUESTION 64

You are teaching a group of occupational medicine trainees about the adverse health effects of noise exposure. One student has a query about noise-induced hearing loss:

Which one of the following types of pathology is noise-induced hearing loss?

a) Conductive hearing loss
b) Sensorineural hearing loss
c) Mixed hearing loss
d) Central hearing loss
e) It can be any of the above

QUESTION 65

You see a 30-year-old baker with a 6-month history of erythema and vesicles on his hands. On examination, there are multiple vesicles and erythematous skin patches, along with some areas of lichenification. There is no evidence of wheals. He describes a pattern of skin disease that worsens at work and improves during holidays. He has no relevant past medical history.

What would be the most appropriate next step in the investigation?

a) Incisional biopsy
b) Patch test
c) Prick test
d) Punch biopsy
e) Skin swabs

QUESTION 66

A 45-year-old site manager at a construction company is responsible for ensuring the safety of the workers on site. During a safety meeting, a new regulation is discussed, which requires the manager to formally identify and evaluate potential hazards that could harm the workers. The manager is unsure which specific legislation mandates this requirement for a risk assessment.

Which legislation introduced the concept of mandatory risk assessment in the workplace?

a) The Health and Safety at Work Act 1974
b) The Management of Health and Safety at Work Regulations 1999
c) The Control of Substances Hazardous to Health Regulations 2002
d) The Personal Protective Equipment at Work Regulations 1992
e) The Workplace (Health, Safety and Welfare) Regulations 1992

QUESTION 67

You are advising a private health clinic that is moving from lower level skin surveillance to a higher level skin surveillance programme following a new case of occupational dermatitis in the workplace.

What is the most appropriate step to be added to the previous health surveillance programme?

a) Informing employees about likely exposures and symptoms to watch out for
b) Increasing the frequency of the previous provisions
c) Instructing employees on how and to whom to report symptoms if they occur
d) Occupational health review of all questionnaires
e) Regular visual skin inspections by a responsible person

QUESTION 68

You are an OH professional reviewing the health surveillance protocols for a company where employees are exposed to whole body vibration (WBV) due to the use of heavy machinery. The company wants to ensure compliance with current regulations and best practices.

Which of the following statements is true regarding health surveillance for employees exposed to whole body vibration?

a) Routine health surveillance is optional for all employees exposed to WBV
b) Health surveillance is not appropriate for WBV
c) Health surveillance for WBV should include routine imaging of the spine to detect early changes

d) An annual checklist for employees exposed to WBV is mandated under UK regulations
e) Health surveillance should focus on early detection of changes in posture

QUESTION 69

You are a newly qualified OHP and have been asked to conduct a medical examination for a group of workers who are exposed to hazardous substances. Your supervisor informs you that the examination must be conducted by an 'appointed doctor' according to statutory requirements.

Which of the following best describes the primary role of an 'appointed doctor'?

a) To provide general medical care to workers
b) To perform specialist care for employees
c) To conduct statutory medical surveillance
d) To provide health and safety advice under COSHH regulations
e) To manage workplace injuries and first aid

QUESTION 70

A construction worker presents with symptoms of carpal tunnel syndrome (CTS). He reports using vibratory tools frequently in his job. A vibration risk assessment performed since his symptoms started shows vibration exposure is kept as low as reasonably practicable.

What is the most appropriate recommendation for his employer to reduce his risk of worsening CTS?

a) Advise the employer to pay for nerve conduction studies
b) Advise the employer to allow more breaks between tasks
c) Advise the employer to conduct an ergonomic assessment
d) Advise the employer to provide wrist splints
e) Advise the employer to redeploy the individual

QUESTION 71

You are a new OHP. You see Mr McDougall, who has given consent for their report to be released, and stated that they do not wish to see their report prior to its dissemination.

What is the recommended best practice in this situation?

a) Do not send the report to either the worker or the referrer if the worker declines to view it
b) Send the report to the referring manager and inform them that it is their responsibility to provide a copy to the worker if requested
c) Send a copy of the report to the worker at the same time as you send it to the referrer
d) Send the report to the referrer and inform the worker that they can request a copy from your company if they change their mind
e) Send the report to the employee for prior viewing anyway

QUESTION 72

You are discussing the role of the Employment Medical Advisory Service (EMAS) with a group of occupational medicine trainees.

Which one of the following is a responsibility of EMAS staff?

a) Provide medical treatment for work-related diseases
b) Provide an occupational health service for organisations that do not have in-house services
c) Provide rehabilitation for people with disabilities under the Equality Act 2010 in employment
d) Conduct statutory medical examinations under the relevant legislation
e) Investigate ill-health reports received under the Reporting of Injuries, Diseases and Dangerous Occurrences Regulations 2013 (RIDDOR)

QUESTION 73

You see a 60-year-old employee for long-term sickness absence. He tells you he does not want to return to work and has handed in his notice. He asks you how long his occupational health notes and report will be retained by the department. Reports in the department are retained in compliance with General Data Protection Regulations (GDPR).

What is the most appropriate retention period for his occupational health reports?

a) 40 years
b) His employment period plus 6 years
c) Indefinitely, in case of future legal claims
d) Until his 75th birthday
e) Until his retirement age

QUESTION 74

A 30-year-old healthcare worker has their blood tested for hepatitis B immunity status. Their results are as follows:

HBsAg (hepatitis B surface antigen): Negative

HBsAb (hepatitis B surface antibody): Positive

HBcAb (hepatitis B core antibody): Positive

How best should these results be interpreted, and what action is needed?

a) The individual has an active hepatitis B infection and needs treatment
b) The individual is immune due to vaccination, and no further action is required
c) The individual has recovered from a past hepatitis B infection and is protected; no vaccine is needed
d) The individual is not immune and is at risk for hepatitis B; a vaccine is needed
e) The individual is a carrier of hepatitis B and should be monitored closely

QUESTION 75

A 45-year-old office worker is recovering from long Covid and is preparing to return to work. The company's policy allows for a phased return to work (RTW) with a maximum duration of 4 weeks.

What is the most appropriate advice for managing RTW in employees recovering from long Covid?

a) The four-week phased RTW plan is typically sufficient for individuals with long Covid

b) Individuals recovering from long Covid generally need a longer phased RTW period than the standard 4 weeks
c) Employees with long Covid should resume full-time work as soon as their symptoms improve
d) A phased RTW is unnecessary for people recovering from long Covid
e) The employee should delay returning to work for at least 6 months after recovering from long Covid symptoms

QUESTION 76

You are an OH professional reviewing a risk assessment at a bottling factory. You note that static monitoring has shown high noise levels in certain areas. Workers move through various roles throughout their shifts, including assembly lines.

Which of the following is the most appropriate method for accurately measuring an employee's exposure to noise over a work shift?

a) Sound level meter
b) Dosimeter
c) Photometer
d) Personal noise alarm
e) Accelerometer

QUESTION 77

You are teaching a group of diploma students about the effects of radiation in the workplace. One student asks you what the 'effective dose' means.

What is the most appropriate answer?

a) Is the concentration of energy deposited in tissue as a result of an exposure to ionising radiation
b) Takes into account the concentration of energy deposited in tissue as a result of an exposure to ionising radiation and addresses the relative harm of each that the type of radiation has on that tissue
c) Takes into account the concentration of energy deposited in tissue as a result of an exposure to ionising radiation, the relative harm level of the radiation, and the sensitivities of each organ to radiation

d) Takes into account the concentration of energy deposited in tissue as a result of an exposure to ionising radiation, the relative harm level of the radiation, and the sensitivities of each organ to radiation specific to children
e) Takes into account the concentration of energy deposited in tissue as a result of an exposure to ionising radiation, the relative harm level of the radiation, and the sensitivities of each organ to radiation specific to the foetus

QUESTION 78

Which one of the following regulations is not part of the 'Six Pack' regulations in the UK?

a) Management of Health and Safety at Work Regulations 1999
b) Reporting of Injuries, Diseases and Dangerous Occurrences Regulations 2013
c) Personal Protective Equipment Regulations 2002
d) Workplace (Health, Safety and Welfare) Regulations 1992
e) Manual Handling Operations Regulations 1992

QUESTION 79

A 50-year-old man undergoes a routine hearing test as part of his occupational health surveillance. The audiogram shows that the difference of the sum of the hearing levels at 1, 2, 3 and 4 kHz for both ears is greater than 40 dB.

What is the most appropriate next step in management?

a) No action, place back into normal surveillance
b) Refer back to GP/ENT for consideration of atypical noise-induced hearing loss
c) Refer back to GP/ENT to exclude acoustic neuroma
d) Refer for otoacoustic emission tests
e) Repeat the audiogram in 6 months

QUESTION 80

Which of the following statements most accurately reflects the challenges faced by younger workers during and after the Covid-19 pandemic, compared to older workers?

a) Younger workers were less likely to be furloughed during the pandemic
b) Younger workers are more likely to exhibit presenteeism
c) Younger workers are more at risk of long-term unemployment
d) Younger workers are more likely to report mental health concerns to their employer
e) Younger workers are less likely to work in sectors affected by the Covid-19 pandemic

ANSWERS to Mock exam 1

QUESTION 1

You take a group of occupational health (OH) trainees on a workplace visit to a workshop where paint spraying with isocyanate-containing paint is used. One worker shows you his test results which say that 'di-amines are not present in his urine'.

A student asks you what type of test this is. What is the most appropriate answer?

The answer is: b) Biological monitoring

The test results indicating 'di-amines are not present in urine' reflect biological monitoring, as this type of test measures the levels of chemicals or their metabolites in biological samples to assess exposure to hazardous substances; in this case, isocyanates.

Biological monitoring involves measuring the levels of chemicals or their metabolites in biological samples, such as urine, blood or breath. The test for di-amines in urine falls under this category, as it directly measures the metabolite of isocyanates to assess exposure.

In contrast, biological effect monitoring is the measurement of the biological effects resulting from absorption of chemicals. An example of this would be measurement of protein in urine of workers exposed to cadmium, to check their kidney function.

A drug test is used to detect the presence of illegal or controlled substances in the body. The test for di-amines in urine is related to occupational exposure to isocyanates, not drug use.

Health screening is a broader term that typically refers to tests or checks used to identify potential health issues in asymptomatic individuals. The specific test for di-amines is not a general health screening but rather a targeted test for occupational exposure.

Health surveillance is an ongoing process involving regular health checks and monitoring to detect early signs of work-related ill health. While biological monitoring can be part of health surveillance, the specific test for di-amines in urine is more accurately described as biological monitoring.

Sources:
- www.hsl.gov.uk/media/1664371/employers.pdf
- Sadhra, S., Bray, A.J. and Boorman, S. (eds) (2022) *Oxford Handbook of Occupational Health*, 3rd edition

QUESTION 2

You are assessing an employee who has developed skin lesions after prolonged dioxin exposure. On examination, there are open comedones on the cheeks.

Which of the following is the most likely diagnosis?

The answer is: d) Chloracne

Chloracne is a specific skin condition caused by exposure to poly-halogenated aromatic hydrocarbons, such as chlorinated dibenzodioxins. It typically presents with open pale comedones and cysts on the face and neck.

Source: Sadhra, S., Bray, A.J. and Boorman, S. (eds) (2022) *Oxford Handbook of Occupational Health*, 3rd edition

QUESTION 3

A construction worker who recently had surgery for Dupuytren's disease is preparing to return to work. He is concerned about the possibility of his symptoms recurring due to his exposure to vibrating tools.

What is the most appropriate advice for him regarding his return to work?

The answer is: b) There is no existing evidence indicating that using vibrating tools at work raises the risk of symptoms returning

Current evidence does not support the idea that exposure to vibrating tools increases the likelihood of symptom recurrence after surgery for Dupuytren's disease. However, recurrence of symptoms is relatively common after surgery or collagenase treatment, regardless of vibration exposure.

Source: www.som.org.uk/sites/som.org.uk/files/Dupuytrens_Disease_and_work_with_hand-held_vibrating_tools.pdf

QUESTION 4

You are the occupational health (OH) practitioner for an ambulance service. A staff member was exposed to both hepatitis B and hepatitis C in the line of duty and has attended your clinic for post-exposure counselling. She asks when her first test for hepatitis B and C will be.

What is the most appropriate response?

The answer is: c) 6 weeks after exposure

In practice, a department may take a blood sample immediately after the incident and save it; the blood will only be tested later if doubts are raised as to whether the person contracted the blood-borne virus through the event, or whether it was pre-existing.

Testing for hepatitis B (HBV) and hepatitis C (HCV) infection should be performed at 6 weeks, 3 months and 6 months following exposure. If the worker has been adequately vaccinated against HBV, only HCV testing is necessary. The initial testing at 6 weeks helps detect any early signs of infection, with further testing done to definitively confirm or exclude the infection.

Source: https://assets.publishing.service.gov.uk/media/5d948c36e5274a2fb1019c1a/Guidance_on_management_of_potential_exposure_to_blood__2_.pdf

QUESTION 5

You are working with a renovation firm reviewing the requirements for maintaining the asbestos health records for their operatives. The Human Resources department is unclear about how long these records need to be kept for.

For how long must asbestos health records be kept?

The answer is: d) 40 years

Statutory health surveillance may be needed under COSHH, Noise, Vibration, Lead, Asbestos and Ionising Radiations Regulations. Employers must maintain a basic health record containing employee details, exposure information, surveillance conducted, tester's name and fitness outcomes. These records are not confidential and can be managed by employers, while detailed clinical records remain confidential and require consent for disclosure. Statutory health records must be retained for 40 years (30 years for ionising radiation), though clinical records generally do not need to be kept as long unless there is a specific reason.

Source: www.fom.ac.uk/media-events/news/guidance/guidance-on-the-general-data-protection-regulation

QUESTION 6

You are a medical educator teaching a class about occupational health. During the lecture, you present a case study about a 58-year-old male who has been diagnosed with lung cancer after working for 30 years in an environment with heavy asbestos exposure. The class discusses various carcinogens and their International Agency for Research on Cancer (IARC) classifications.

Which IARC classification indicates that an agent is known to be carcinogenic to humans?

The answer is: a) Group 1

In the context of IARC classifications:

Group 1: "Carcinogenic to humans". There is enough evidence to conclude that it can cause cancer in humans.

Group 2A: "Probably carcinogenic to humans". There is strong evidence that it can cause cancer in humans, but at present it is not conclusive.

Group 2B: "Possibly carcinogenic to humans". There is some evidence that it can cause cancer in humans, but at present it is far from conclusive.

Group 3: "Unclassifiable as to carcinogenicity in humans". There is no evidence at present that it causes cancer in humans.

Answers to Mock exam 1

Group 4: "Probably not carcinogenic to humans". There is strong evidence that it does not cause cancer in humans.

Source: https://monographs.iarc.who.int/agents-classified-by-the-iarc

QUESTION 7

A 45-year-old employee is seeking reasonable adjustments at work due to a chronic condition. The employee has not received a formal medical diagnosis but reports significant limitations in daily activities due to pain and fatigue. The employer is unsure whether the employee qualifies for reasonable adjustments under the law, given the lack of a specific diagnosis.

When determining whether this employee qualifies for reasonable adjustments under disability legislation, which of the following is most relevant to consider?

The answer is: d) The effect of the impairment

To qualify for accommodations, it is the effect of an impairment that matters, not the need for a medically diagnosed cause. It is not necessary to categorise the impairment as either physical or mental, as its effects may be complex and could involve both physical and mental aspects. Additionally, physical effects might originate from mental impairments, and vice versa.

Source: Hobson, J. and Smedley, J. (eds) (2019) *Fitness for Work: the medical aspects*, 6th edition. Oxford University Press

QUESTION 8

You are an occupational physician assessing a 55-year-old factory worker who has severe chronic obstructive pulmonary disease (COPD). Despite his condition, he believes he can continue his physically demanding job without any changes or restrictions. You are concerned that his severe COPD significantly limits his ability to safely perform his duties and believe that he should be redeployed to a sedentary role. During the assessment, the worker strongly expresses his desire to remain in his current role without modifications and resists any suggestion of changing his job responsibilities.

What is the most appropriate action to take?

The answer is: c) Document the worker's views but explain your opinion that redeployment is needed

Good medical practice involves respecting a worker's right to be involved in decisions about their care, including job placement. While it is important to consider the worker's views and document them, an occupational health physician must provide an impartial recommendation based on medical evidence to ensure the worker's safety and health. In this case, given the worker's severe COPD, it is not safe for him to continue in a physically demanding role. Redeployment to a sedentary role is needed, and this should be communicated clearly to the worker while acknowledging his preferences.

If you opine that he is fit for work without adjustments, respecting his wishes: this disregards the medical risks posed by the worker's severe COPD and does not provide an evidence-based recommendation.

Recommending medical retirement does not consider the possibility of the worker continuing to work in a role suited to his medical condition, and unnecessarily limits his options.

Ignoring the worker's preferences and speaking to the manager about redeploying him to a different role fails to involve the worker in decision-making and does not respect his right to be part of the process or the process of consent.

While respecting autonomy is important, an occupational health physician must provide an impartial, evidence-based recommendation that ensures health and safety.

QUESTION 9

You are running a careers session for doctors interested in occupational medicine. During the session, a doctor asks about the requirements for conducting medical examinations for seafarers.

Which one of the following types of doctor are authorised to carry out seafarer medical examinations?

The answer is: a) Maritime and Coastguard Agency (MCA) Approved Doctors

Medical practitioners approved by the Maritime and Coastguard Agency (MCA) are authorised to conduct medical examinations for seafarers. These practitioners, referred to as Approved Doctors (ADs), are appointed under Merchant Shipping legislation for a statutory period, typically one year.

Source: https://assets.publishing.service.gov.uk/media/5f10af97d3bf7f5babafec43/Approved_Doctors_Manual_July_2020.pdf

QUESTION 10

You are assisting an employer in reviewing their guidance on procedures for noise health surveillance. The current guidance advises employees to wait 10 hours after exposure to loud noise before undergoing surveillance audiometry. However, you identify that this recommendation does not align with best practice, which aims to minimise the influence of temporary threshold shifts (TTS) on audiometry results.

How should the guidance be amended to align with best practice for noise health surveillance?

The answer is: d) Change the waiting period to 16 hours after noise exposure

This aligns with best practice recommendations to minimise the influence of temporary threshold shifts (TTS) on audiometry results.

TTS are threshold shifts in hearing that recover to baseline levels in the hours, days or weeks following exposure to noise.

To minimise the influence of TTS and conduct accurate hearing tests, it is recommended workers should avoid loud noise or sound for at least 16 hours before surveillance audiometry.

Source: Sadhra, S., Bray, A.J. and Boorman, S. (eds) (2022) *Oxford Handbook of Occupational Health*, 3rd edition

QUESTION 11

You are reviewing the occupational health risks associated with welding.

Which one of the following infections are welders at an increased risk of developing due to their occupation?

The answer is: c) *Streptococcus pneumoniae*

Welders are at increased risk of developing *Streptococcus pneumoniae* infections, including pneumococcal pneumonia, due to their exposure to metal fumes. Metal fumes can impair lung defences, increasing susceptibility to respiratory infections. This is why vaccination against *Streptococcus pneumoniae* is recommended for welders to mitigate this occupational risk. The other listed infections are not specifically associated with welding exposure.

QUESTION 12

You are reviewing a case involving a 38-year-old welder who reports a sudden onset of eye pain, tearing, and redness after working on a welding project. The worker describes the sensation as feeling like he has "sand in the eye" and mentions a high sensitivity to light.

What is the most likely cause of this worker's symptoms?

The answer is: b) Ultraviolet (UV) radiation

The worker's symptoms are characteristic of 'arc eye' or 'welder's eye', which is caused by exposure to UV radiation emitted during welding. UV radiation can cause damage to the cornea and conjunctiva, leading to symptoms such as pain, redness, tearing, and the sensation of sand in the eye, as well as photophobia (abnormal sensitivity to light). Given the context of the worker's exposure to welding activities and the onset of these symptoms, UV radiation is the most likely cause.

Chemical exposure can cause eye irritation and pain. Moreover, the worker's symptoms arose after welding, which is not directly associated with chemical exposure in this context.

Dust exposure is also less specific to the activity of welding, making this a less likely cause.

Infrared radiation from welding can cause thermal injuries to the eyes, but these injuries typically do not present with the described symptoms.

Bacterial conjunctivitis can cause redness, tearing and discomfort, but it does not typically cause an immediate onset of pain or a sensation of "sand in the eye" following welding activities. Additionally, there would generally be other signs of infection, such as discharge, which were not reported in this case.

Answers to Mock exam 1

QUESTION 13

A 55-year-old woman presents with numbness, tingling and pain in her hands, which worsens at night. On examination, you suspect carpal tunnel syndrome (CTS).

Which one of the following is a constitutional risk factor for developing carpal tunnel syndrome?

The answer is: a) Diabetes

Diabetes is a well-recognised constitutional risk factor for CTS. Other risk factors include a high BMI, rheumatoid arthritis, and conditions affecting nerve function. These factors can predispose individuals to increased pressure on the median nerve in the carpal tunnel, leading to CTS symptoms. Low BMI, alcohol use, poor hand hygiene, and a sedentary lifestyle are not direct constitutional risk factors for CTS.

Source: www.som.org.uk/sites/som.org.uk/files/Carpal_tunnel_syndrome_and_work_with_hand-held_vibrating_tools_Jan2022.pdf

QUESTION 14

A 45-year-old office worker was scheduled for health surveillance required by their employer. However, the employee did not attend the scheduled appointment. As an independent practitioner, you are considering whether to inform the employer about the missed appointment.

Which one of the following statements is true regarding informing an employer about an employee's failure to attend an appointment?

The answer is: b) Informing the employer about the missed health assessment does not require the employee's consent

Informing the employer about the missed health assessment does not require the employee's consent, as it does not constitute clinical information.

Source: www.fom.ac.uk/wp-content/uploads/GOMP_2017_Web.pdf

QUESTION 15

You are an OH professional advising a healthcare worker (HCW) on the categorisation of their clinical procedures to assess the risk of exposure-prone procedures (EPPs).

Which one of the following is classified as a Category 3 EPP?

The answer is: c) Hysterectomy

The categorisation of EPPs is based on the visibility of the worker's hands during the procedure and the likelihood of injury to the worker's gloved hands, which could result in the worker's blood contaminating the patient's open tissues.

The definition of EPPs covers a wide range of procedures, in which there may be very different levels of risk of bleed-back.

A risk-based categorisation of clinical procedures has been developed, including procedures where there is negligible risk of bleed-back (non-EPP) and three categories of EPPs with increasing risk of bleed-back.

It should be noted that the majority of HCWs do not perform EPPs.

Hysterectomy is a Category 3 EPP, where the fingertips are out of sight for a significant part of the procedure, and there is a distinct risk of injury to the worker's gloved hands, potentially exposing the patient's open tissues to the worker's blood.

Local anaesthetic injection in dentistry is classified as a Category 1 EPP, where the hands and fingertips of the worker are usually visible and outside the body most of the time, and the risk of injury to the worker's gloved hands is slight.

Routine tooth extraction is classified as a Category 2 EPP, where the fingertips may not be visible at all times, but the risk of injury is low and can be quickly addressed if it occurs.

Rigid sigmoidoscopy including biopsy is classified as a non-EPP because the hands and fingertips are visible and outside the patient's body at all times.

Removal of haemorrhoids is classified as a Category 1 EPP, with minimal risk of bleed-back since the hands and fingertips are visible and outside the body most of the time.

Answers to Mock exam 1

Category 3 EPPs carry a higher risk of exposure to the healthcare worker's blood due to the nature of the procedure.

Sources:
- https://assets.publishing.service.gov.uk/media/6627a9b0d29479e036a7e622/integrated-guidance-for-management-of-BBV-in-HCW-April-2024-update.pdf
- https://assets.publishing.service.gov.uk/media/5c40663ae5274a6e4f614dc1/general_surgery_exposure_prone_procedure_epp_categorisation.pdf
- Sadhra, S., Bray, A.J. and Boorman, S. (eds) (2022) *Oxford Handbook of Occupational Health*, 3rd edition

QUESTION 16

You are shadowing at an occupational lung disease clinic. A 50-year-old engineer in the aerospace industry presents with shortness of breath, unexplained coughing, fatigue, weight loss, fever and night sweats. Imaging reveals florid non-caseating granulomatous lung disease.

What is the most likely occupational exposure that would cause his symptoms?

The answer is: a) Beryllium

Beryllium exposure can lead to a condition known as chronic beryllium disease (CBD), which is a rare granulomatous lung disease. The symptoms described (shortness of breath, coughing, fatigue, weight loss, fever and night sweats), and the imaging, are consistent with this condition.

Exposure to cadmium is more typically associated with kidney damage and obstructive lung disease rather than granulomatous lung disease.

Cobalt exposure can cause various lung diseases, but it is less commonly associated with granulomatous lung disease compared to beryllium.

TB can cause granulomatous disease but is not specifically an occupational exposure in the context of the aerospace industry.

Exposure to silica is linked with an increased risk of tuberculosis, which typically has caseating granulomatous disease.

Source: www.ccohs.ca/oshanswers/diseases/beryllium.html

QUESTION 17

An aviary has become aware of a psittacosis outbreak at the local zoo, including an infection in staff. They contact you to help them avoid this affecting their business.

Using the hierarchy of control, which of the following actions is the most effective way to reduce the risk of an outbreak?

The answer is: a) Ensure good ventilation in bird housing

Good ventilation (an engineering control) is the most effective control measure according to the hierarchy of controls.

Ventilation helps to reduce the concentration of airborne pathogens, such as those causing psittacosis, thereby reducing the risk of infection. This approach addresses the problem at the source and controls the environment to prevent the spread of disease.

Good hygiene practices (an administrative control), including handwashing, are important for personal protection and reducing the risk of infection, but do not address the broader issue of airborne pathogen control within the aviary.

While isolating sick birds helps prevent the spread of disease among the flock, it does not address the airborne transmission of pathogens within the aviary. This measure is reactive rather than proactive and does not prevent initial contamination.

Regular cleaning (an administrative control) is important, but high-pressure jet washing can create aerosols that may spread pathogens. Cleaning methods should minimise aerosol generation to avoid inadvertently increasing the risk of exposure.

Wearing protective clothing is important for personal protection but does not control the spread of pathogens in the environment. It is a form of personal protective equipment (PPE) and is less effective compared to engineering controls such as ventilation.

By prioritising good ventilation, the risk of psittacosis outbreaks can be more effectively managed, creating a safer environment for both the birds and the staff.

Sources:
- www.hse.gov.uk/agriculture/assets/docs/psittacosis.pdf
- www.ccohs.ca/oshanswers/hsprograms/hazard/hierarchy_controls.html

Answers to Mock exam 1

QUESTION 18

You are advising a local council that has identified high rates of work-related stress, reducing their employee retention rates. As part of their plan to reduce employee ill health, they have updated their bullying and harassment policy.

Which one of the Health and Safety Executive (HSE) Management Standards does this action address?

The answer is: c) Relationships

The relationships component in the HSE Management Standards framework promotes positive working environments and deals with unacceptable behaviour, directly addressing issues such as bullying and harassment.

There are six areas of work that can have a negative impact on employee health if not properly managed. These are outlined in the Management Standards, along with descriptions of good practice:
- Demands – refers to workload, work patterns and the work environment
- Control – how much say a person has in the way they do their work
- Support – involves the encouragement, sponsorship and resources provided by the organisation, line management and colleagues
- Role – role clarity ensures employees understand their job roles and responsibilities
- Change – how organisational change (large or small) is managed and communicated in the organisation
- Relationships – involves promoting positive working to avoid conflict and dealing with unacceptable behaviour.

Source: www.hse.gov.uk/stress/standards

QUESTION 19

You encounter a 35-year-old baker presenting with symptoms suggestive of occupational asthma.

Which investigation should be pursued next to establish a diagnosis?

The answer is: c) Serial peak flows

Serial peak expiratory flow (PEF) recordings are the investigative method of choice for suspected cases of occupational asthma and should ideally be conducted early, prior to starting maintenance therapy, and while the patient is still exposed to potential allergens at work.

The patient should first be instructed in basic PEF technique by a suitably qualified professional.

The best of three PEF readings should be recorded every 2 hours during waking time. Measurements should be continued at home and at work.

Reading should continue for a period of at least 4 weeks, including a period of at least 1 week away from work.

Sources:
- www.brit-thoracic.org.uk/quality-improvement/clinical-statements/occupational-asthma
- Sadhra, S., Bray, A.J. and Boorman, S. (eds) (2022) *Oxford Handbook of Occupational Health*, 3rd edition

QUESTION 20

You are an OH doctor for a local charity. An employee who has a diagnosis of secondary progressive multiple sclerosis (MS) and now needs to use a wheelchair, requests that a lift be installed so she can access the upper floors of the workplace where she works. After conducting a cost-analysis exercise, the employer finds that installing a lift would be unaffordable for the business. The employer seeks your advice on how to proceed in compliance with the Equality Act 2010.

What is the most appropriate advice to give the employer?

The answer is: b) Suggest that the employee's request is denied but explore modifying her role so she can work on the ground floor

The Equality Act 2010 requires employers to make reasonable adjustments for disabled employees.

What is reasonable depends on each situation. The employer must consider carefully whether the adjustment:
- will remove or reduce the disadvantage – the employer should talk with the person and not make assumptions
- is practical to make
- is affordable
- could harm the health and safety of others.

Answers to Mock exam 1

The Equality Act requires reasonable adjustments, not necessarily fulfilling every request if it is not feasible. Installing a lift that is unaffordable for the business may not be considered reasonable.

If the cost of installing a lift is too high, the employer must find other feasible solutions, such as relocating a work area to the ground floor, to ensure she can perform her job effectively.

While working from home might be a temporary solution, suggesting it permanently without exploring other reasonable adjustments in the workplace could be seen as exclusionary and not a balanced approach.

While the Access to Work Scheme can provide support, it does not replace the employer's legal obligation to make reasonable adjustments. Suggesting this alone without providing direct adjustments is not sufficient.

While redeployment can be considered, it should not be the first or only solution. The employer must first attempt to make reasonable adjustments to her current role.

Source: www.gov.uk/reasonable-adjustments-for-disabled-workers

QUESTION 21

You are evaluating a 60-year-old gardener who has been referred for consideration of ill-health retirement due to long Covid. During the examination, you notice a 2 cm lesion on his face with a rolled, pearly edge and central ulceration.

What is the most likely occupational exposure that could cause this type of lesion?

The answer is: c) Ultraviolet (UV) radiation

The lesion described – a 2 cm facial lesion with a rolled, pearly edge and central ulceration – is characteristic of basal cell carcinoma (BCC). BCC is commonly associated with prolonged exposure to UV radiation from the sun. Gardeners, who spend significant time outdoors, are at increased risk of developing BCC due to chronic sun exposure.

Anthrax can cause skin lesions, but these lesions typically present as a black eschar rather than a pearly, ulcerative lesion.

Fungal infections such as tinea typically cause ring-shaped, scaly lesions, not a pearly-edged ulcer.

Exposure to latex can lead to allergic reactions or contact dermatitis, but these do not present as a pearly-edged ulcerative lesion.

While certain plants such as celery can cause photodermatitis or allergic reactions, they do not typically cause lesions with the described characteristics of BCC.

QUESTION 22

You are speaking to a group of trainee occupational physicians about the long-term effects of chemical exposures, focusing on vinyl chloride monomer (VCM), a substance used in the production of polyvinyl chloride (PVC).

Which of the following is a long-term health effect associated with chronic exposure to VCM?

The answer is: e) all of the above

These conditions were first identified in association with historically high exposures to VCM but are unlikely to arise from present-day working practices due to strict control of exposure.

VCM is a colourless gas with a sweet odour, primarily used in the production of PVC. Inhalation is the main exposure route.

Chronic VCM exposure has been associated with several long-term health effects, including the following:
- Acro-osteolysis: decalcification of terminal phalanges, leading to pseudo-clubbing, scleroderma and Raynaud's disease, which can occur independently. Symptoms may improve with removal from exposure.
- Angiosarcoma of the liver: a rare tumour with a long latency period.
- Non-cirrhotic portal fibrosis: associated with historical high exposures to VCM.
- Hepatocellular carcinoma: identified as a health risk by the International Agency for Research on Cancer in 2012.

Source: https://www.hse.gov.uk/pubns/ms32.pdf

QUESTION 23

A 43-year-old care worker comes to you with a one-year history of fibromyalgia. She has found it increasingly difficult to concentrate due to 'brain fog' and continues to find shift work difficult because of fatigue. She has not seen occupational health previously, and no action has been taken at work to date. She wishes to be considered for ill-health retirement.

Which one of the following is the most appropriate next step to be considered in her management?

The answer is: a) Adjustments

The consideration and implementation of adjustments is the most appropriate next step.

Employers have a duty to make reasonable adjustments for employees with disabilities, such as fibromyalgia. Adjustments might include modifying her duties, altering her work schedule, or providing support to help manage symptoms such as brain fog and fatigue.

Ill-health retirement is a significant and final step that should be considered only after exploring all other reasonable accommodations and adjustments.

Redeployment should be considered if adjustments are not feasible, but the first step should be to try to accommodate her in her current role.

Referring to a senior colleague could be part of the process, but it is not a direct management step for her condition.

Advising her to stay on sick leave until symptom resolution is not appropriate. Fibromyalgia is a chronic condition without a definitive resolution, making long-term sick leave impractical as a primary management step.

QUESTION 24

You see an employee in clinic who works with 3D printers. He tells you that he thinks working with this machine has caused his diagnosis of psoriasis.

In evaluating whether an occupational exposure is linked to a particular disease, you are considering the Bradford Hill criteria.

Which of the following best describes the use of the criterion 'Analogy'?

The answer is: b) Determining if similar exposures are known to cause the disease in other settings or populations

The Analogy criterion involves evaluating whether similar exposures or conditions have been shown to cause the disease in other contexts or populations. This criterion helps to strengthen the case for causation by demonstrating that if other analogous exposures are known to cause the disease, then the same mechanism might be at work in the current situation. This comparison can provide additional support for the hypothesis that the occupational exposure in question may also be causative.

The Bradford Hill criteria used to determine causation:
- *Strength of association*: examines the magnitude of the relationship between exposure and disease. A stronger association (e.g. a high relative risk or odds ratio) lends more weight to the causal inference. If the exposure is strongly linked to the disease, it supports the likelihood of a causal relationship.
- *Temporality*: refers to whether the exposure precedes the onset of the disease. For a causal relationship, the exposure must occur before the disease develops. This is a fundamental criterion because if the disease occurs before the exposure, causation cannot be established.
- *Dose–response relationship*: assesses whether increasing levels of exposure result in a corresponding increase in the risk of the disease. A clear dose–response relationship supports causation, as it suggests that higher exposures lead to higher risks of disease, demonstrating a biological gradient.
- *Analogy*: involves comparing the exposure–disease relationship to similar known relationships in other contexts. If similar exposures have been shown to cause the same or similar diseases elsewhere, it supports the likelihood that the exposure in question might also be causative.
- *Consistency*: refers to whether the association between exposure and disease is observed across different studies, populations and settings. A consistent finding across various studies and conditions strengthens the evidence for a causal relationship.
- *Coherence*: examines whether the association makes sense within the broader context of existing knowledge about the disease and exposure. It checks if the findings are consistent with the known biology and other evidence related to the disease.

Answers to Mock exam 1

- *Specificity*: looks at whether the exposure is associated with a specific disease and not with other unrelated diseases. A high degree of specificity suggests that the exposure–disease relationship is causal, though this criterion is less commonly met in complex exposures.
- *Experiment*: involves evidence from experiments or interventions. If altering the exposure (e.g. through control measures or treatment) leads to changes in the incidence or prevalence of the disease, it supports the causal relationship. Experimental evidence can strengthen the case for causation.

Each of these criteria provides a different angle of evidence for evaluating causality, and collectively they help in assessing whether a particular exposure causes a disease.

QUESTION 25

Mr Smith is a manager working in the nuclear industry where many workers are industrial radiographers. Mr Smith is concerned about the potential health risks associated with radiation exposure and wants to ensure that all staff are correctly designated as classified workers where appropriate.

Under the Ionising Radiations Regulations 2017, which one of the following is true regarding the designation of classified workers?

The answer is: b) It is the duty of the employer to designate an individual as a classified worker

Under the Ionising Radiations Regulations 2017, the employer is responsible for deciding whether to designate an individual as a classified worker, based on their potential exposure to ionising radiation. Employers may consult a radiation protection adviser to help inform this decision, but the responsibility lies with the employer, not the adviser or the worker themselves.

Source: www.hse.gov.uk/radiation/ionising/doses/designation.htm

QUESTION 26

An employer is evaluating dust exposure in the workplace and needs to understand the term 'inhalable dust' to better assess potential health risks.

Which one of the following is the definition of 'inhalable dust'?

The answer is: b) Dust that can enter the nose and mouth during breathing, including particles that may cause damage to the upper respiratory tract

Inhalable dust diameters range from 0.05 μm to 200.0 μm. They are defined as the fraction of total airborne particles that are inhaled through the nose and/or mouth. These dusts tend to get trapped in the nose, mouth, throat or upper respiratory tract, where they can cause damage. An example includes wood dust.

Respirable dust diameters range from 0.05 μm to 10.0 μm. They are defined as the fraction of airborne particles that penetrate to the lower gas-exchange region of the lung (alveolar region). These dusts can build up in the air spaces in the lungs and can lead to lung damage. An example includes silica.

Source: www.hse.gov.uk/dust/assets/docs/eh44.pdf

QUESTION 27

You are the lead physician responsible for an OH service at a large manufacturing company. The company deals with hazardous materials and heavy machinery. During a recent safety audit, you identified several gaps in the company's first aid provisions, including inadequate first aid kits and a lack of trained first aid personnel.

Which would be the best action to take next?

The answer is: b) Advise the employer on the specific first aid requirements and the need to address the identified gaps

As the lead physician responsible for the OH service, you can advise the employer on their legal and practical obligations regarding first aid provisions, especially given the presence of hazardous materials and heavy machinery. While the responsibility for providing first aid lies with the employer, your role includes ensuring that the employer is aware of their responsibilities and that adequate first aid arrangements are in place and properly monitored.

Directly implementing first aid training and purchasing the necessary first aid supplies is not appropriate as it oversteps the advisory role and the duty remains with the employer.

Reporting the company to the HSE for failing to meet first aid standards is a drastic step that should only be taken if the employer fails to address the concerns after being properly advised.

Arranging external first aid providers is outside the scope of the OH service's responsibilities, and bypasses the employer's duty.

Taking no action neglects the proactive role expected of an OH service to advise and ensure proper first aid arrangements are made and monitored.

Source: www.fom.ac.uk/wp-content/uploads/GOMP_2017_Web.pdf

QUESTION 28

An employer at a brewery has conducted a risk assessment before commencing work, which has identified the need for health surveillance. As part of establishing a health surveillance programme, the employer asks you about the primary purpose of health surveillance.

What is the most appropriate answer?

The answer is: e) To detect adverse health effects at an early stage

Health surveillance primarily aims to detect adverse health effects early among employees exposed to occupational hazards. This early detection allows for timely intervention to prevent further harm and implement necessary adjustments to the work environment or job roles.

Health surveillance focuses on early detection rather than formal diagnosis, which typically involves more extensive medical assessments.

While health surveillance indirectly assesses the effectiveness of control measures and the accuracy of risk assessments by monitoring health outcomes, its primary purpose is not specifically to check control measures but to monitor and protect employee health.

Health surveillance is not a form of control.

Source: www.hse.gov.uk/health-surveillance/manage-the-risk.htm

QUESTION 29

You are an OH professional conducting a workplace assessment for a large corporate office. Part of your evaluation includes ensuring that the lighting in the office is adequate for the tasks performed by the staff, which mostly involve computer work and reading documents.

What is the recommended average illuminance (lux) level for an office environment to ensure safe and effective work performance?

The answer is: b) 200–500 lux

According to guidelines, the recommended average illuminance level for an office environment is between 200 and 500 lux. This level of lighting is necessary to ensure that employees can see details clearly without causing visual fatigue, which is crucial for tasks involving reading, writing and computer use. Lower lighting levels might be suitable for less detailed work or circulation routes, but offices require a higher standard to maintain a comfortable and efficient working environment.

Sources:
- www.hse.gov.uk/pubns/priced/hsg38.pdf
- Sadhra, S., Bray, A.J. and Boorman, S. (eds) (2022) *Oxford Handbook of Occupational Health*, 3rd edition

QUESTION 30

A construction worker has been using a vibrating hand tool for the past five years. Recently, he has started experiencing symptoms such as numbness and tingling in his fingers. During your assessment, you review the workplace safety guidelines and vibration exposure levels.

What is generally accepted to be the 'no harm level' of exposure when working with vibrating handheld tools?

The answer is: b) 1 m/sec^2

A vibration exposure level of 1 m/sec^2 is widely accepted as the 'no harm' level. This threshold is used to indicate an exposure level below which it is generally believed that the risk of developing hand arm vibration syndrome (HAVS) is minimal.

Source: www.som.org.uk/sites/som.org.uk/files/HAVS_Guidance_from_SOM_v16.pdf

Answers to Mock exam 1

QUESTION 31

A pregnant worker in an organisation has been exposed to a risk that could potentially harm her or her unborn child. After assessing the situation, the employer finds that they are unable to control or remove the risk.

What should be the best next steps to ensure the worker's health and safety?

The answer is: b) Offer suitable alternative work that is appropriate for the pregnant worker on the same terms and conditions

When a significant risk to a pregnant worker or her child is identified and cannot be controlled or removed, the first step is to adjust the working conditions or hours to avoid the risk. If this is not feasible, the next step is to offer suitable alternative work, which should be appropriate for the pregnant worker or new mother and maintain the same terms and conditions, including pay, as per the Employment Rights Act 1996. If suitable alternative work cannot be provided, the worker should be suspended on paid leave to protect her health and safety and that of her child.

Sources:
- www.hse.gov.uk/mothers/employer/welfare-rights.htm
- Sadhra, S., Bray, A.J. and Boorman, S. (eds) (2022) *Oxford Handbook of Occupational Health*, 3rd edition

QUESTION 32

You are reviewing the occupational health risks associated with sewage exposure.

Which of the following infections are sewage workers at an increased risk of developing due to their occupation?

The answer is: a) Hepatitis A virus

Sewage workers are at increased risk of hepatitis A virus infection due to its faecal–oral transmission route. Hepatitis A can be present in contaminated water and sewage, and exposure through contact with faecal matter increases the risk of infection.

Source: www.hse.gov.uk/construction/healthrisks/hazardous-substances/harmful-micro-organisms/hepatitis-a.htm

QUESTION 33

A company is seeking information on national trends in work-related ill health to better understand the risks in their industry. They are directed to a surveillance scheme specifically designed to monitor the incidence of work-related health conditions in the UK.

Which of the following surveillance schemes has the primary aim of monitoring the incidence and trends in work-related ill health?

The answer is: b) The Health and Occupation Research (THOR) network

The THOR network is a surveillance scheme with the primary aim of monitoring the incidence and trends of work-related ill health in the UK.

While the LFS collects data on employment and health, it is a general survey and not specifically designed to monitor trends in work-related ill health.

WERS focuses on employment relations and workplace practices, not specifically on work-related ill health.

EWCS collects data on working conditions across Europe but is not focused solely on monitoring work-related ill-health trends in the UK.

The National Health Service (NHS) Patient Safety Alert System focuses on patient safety issues within healthcare settings and is not designed to monitor work-related ill health.

Source: https://sites.manchester.ac.uk/thor

QUESTION 34

You see a 29-year-old welder who has been referred for frequent, short sickness absences. On further enquiry she describes fever, shivering and headache, and malaise that she feels occurs in the evening after she is at work. She has not needed any treatment for these symptoms, which she has attributed to viral illness. She has no other past medical history.

What is the most likely diagnosis?

The answer is: c) Metal fume fever

The patient's symptoms of fever, shivering, headache and malaise occurring after being exposed to welding fumes at work are consistent with metal fume fever, a common issue for welders exposed to metal fumes.

COPD is a chronic condition characterised by persistent respiratory symptoms, not typically associated with acute, short-lived episodes of fever and malaise that resolve without treatment.

While influenza could cause fever, shivering, headache and malaise, it is typically more severe, lasts longer, and is not closely linked to specific work exposures.

Occupational asthma presents with respiratory symptoms such as wheezing and shortness of breath, rather than fever and malaise.

Welder's lung involves metal deposition in the lungs and typically does not present with acute, flu-like symptoms.

Source: www.hse.gov.uk/welding/health-risks-welding.htm

QUESTION 35

You have been asked to see a 52-year-old personal assistant with sporadic wheezy episodes whilst at work.

What is the next practical step you should take?

The answer is: b) Take a detailed history

In this scenario, taking a detailed history should come before a workplace inspection. You cannot request further information without his expressed consent and this may not be appropriate at this stage. Requesting investigations would not be your role – this would be down to his treating physician, i.e. the GP or a specialist.

QUESTION 36

Researchers are interested in understanding the relationship between past occupational exposure and the development of a disease with a long latency period.

Which type of study design is most appropriate for investigating this?

The answer is: c) Case–control study

Case–control study: this study design is ideal for investigating diseases with a long latency period. In a case–control study, researchers identify individuals with the disease (cases) and compare them to those without the disease (controls), then look retrospectively at their exposure histories. This method is efficient for studying rare diseases or those that take many years to develop, as it allows for the assessment of past exposures without the need for long follow-up periods.

Cross-sectional study: this design measures exposure and disease status at a single point in time, making it unsuitable for studying the relationship between past exposures and diseases that develop over many years.

Ecological study: an ecological study examines exposure and outcome data at the population level rather than focusing on individual histories, which is not ideal for exploring the detailed exposure history required in cases of long latency diseases.

Prospective cohort study: while a prospective cohort study is useful for studying the incidence of disease, it requires long-term follow-up and is less efficient for diseases with long latency periods compared to a case–control study.

Randomised controlled trial: this design is typically used for testing the effectiveness of interventions rather than for investigating the relationship between past exposures and the development of diseases with long latency periods.

Source: https://casp-uk.net/news/what-is-a-case-control-study

QUESTION 37

You meet with unions at a construction company. They want to talk to you about the health effects of diesel exhaust fumes, to which they feel they are heavily exposed. They are particularly concerned about the risk of cancer.

What is the cancer most associated with diesel fumes?

The answer is: c) Lung

Large populations are exposed to diesel exhaust fumes in everyday life, whether through their occupation or through the ambient air. People are exposed not only to motor vehicle exhausts but also to exhausts from other diesel engines, including from other modes of transport (e.g. diesel trains and ships) and from power generators.

The International Agency for Research on Cancer (IARC) concludes that there is sufficient evidence in humans for the carcinogenicity of diesel exhaust fumes.

Answers to Mock exam 1

The Working Group found that diesel exhaust fumes are a cause of lung cancer (sufficient evidence) and also noted a positive association (limited evidence) with an increased risk of bladder cancer.

NB: although occupational exposure to diesel engine exhaust emissions is known to increase risk of cancer, there is no direct evidence of an increased risk from lower-level environmental exposures.

Sources:
- www.iarc.who.int/wp-content/uploads/2018/07/pr213_E.pdf
- Sadhra, S., Bray, A.J. and Boorman, S. (eds) (2022) *Oxford Handbook of Occupational Health*, 3rd edition

QUESTION 38

You are conducting an OH assessment for a 20-year-old employee recently diagnosed with relapsing–remitting multiple sclerosis (MS) who has experienced complete remission since diagnosis.

What is the most appropriate advice to provide regarding the Equality Act?

The answer is: c) She is covered by the Equality Act immediately upon her diagnosis

Under the Equality Act 2010, individuals diagnosed with MS are protected from discrimination and entitled to reasonable adjustments in the workplace from the moment of diagnosis, regardless of whether they currently have symptoms or are in remission.

The Act states that a person who has cancer, HIV infection or multiple sclerosis (MS) is protected by the Act from the point of diagnosis.

Sources:
- www.equalityhumanrights.com/equality/equality-act-2010/your-rights-under-equality-act-2010/disability-discrimination
- Sadhra, S., Bray, A.J. and Boorman, S. (eds) (2022) *Oxford Handbook of Occupational Health*, 3rd edition

QUESTION 39

You see a 56-year-old tree surgeon who has been referred with numbness and tingling in both hands and episodic blanching of his fingers associated with cold weather. You take a history and examine him, and take his blood pressure. You examine his grip strength and check sensation of his fingers.

What is the next test that is most appropriate?

The answer is: c) Purdue peg board

This employee is being assessed for HAVS, with Tier 4 health surveillance.

Tier 4 tests include:
- Grip dynamometer
- Purdue peg board
- Monofilament
- Blood pressure

Sources:
- www.som.org.uk/sites/som.org.uk/files/HAVS_Guidance_v1.4.pdf
- www.hse.gov.uk/vibration/assets/docs/havocchealth.pdf

QUESTION 40

Which one of the following entities is primarily responsible for enforcing health and safety law in the UK?

The answer is: b) The Health and Safety Executive (HSE)

Health and safety law is mostly enforced by the HSE or the Local Authority (LA). Responsibility for enforcement depends on the type of workplace; for example, LAs are the main enforcing authority in retail and hotel and catering premises, and the HSE is the main enforcing authority in detention centres and university campuses.

Source: www.hse.gov.uk/simple-health-safety/law/health-safety-law.htm

Answers to Mock exam 1

QUESTION 41

You are collaborating with the safety team to evaluate the outcomes of a recent manual handling risk assessment for a group of warehouse workers. A system of manual handling aids has been introduced to facilitate easier transportation of boxes.

What is the most appropriate next step under manual handling regulations as part of the risk assessment process?

The answer is: c) Review any ongoing sickness absence due to musculoskeletal disease

After implementing manual handling aids, it is critical to ensure that these measures are effective in reducing the risk of injury. Monitoring sickness absence due to musculoskeletal disorders provides direct evidence of whether the interventions are working as intended. This step involves checking accident and ill-health data to identify any trends or issues that persist despite the new measures.

This approach aligns with the continuous improvement principle in health and safety management, ensuring that interventions lead to tangible reductions in risk and promoting a safer working environment. Additionally, regular monitoring and review are essential components of an effective risk management system, ensuring ongoing compliance with regulations and safeguarding worker health.

There is no explicit duty in the Manual Handling Operations Regulations to carry out health surveillance. Implementing a health surveillance programme or a less formal health monitoring system can be beneficial. These systems allow for early reporting, monitoring and investigation of symptoms, which can provide valuable information on the effectiveness of manual handling aids and early detection of manual handling injuries.

Conducting individual risk assessments ensures that the specific risks faced by each worker are identified and addressed, but there is no information in this case to suggest that this is the case. This personalised approach is crucial because manual handling risks can vary significantly between individuals due to factors such as physical capabilities, medical history and job tasks. Individual risk assessments help tailor control measures to the needs of each worker, enhancing safety and compliance with regulations. However, this step might be more appropriate as an initial measure rather than a follow-up after implementing handling aids.

Regularly reviewing the risk assessment, e.g. on an annual basis, is a standard part of the risk management process. This review ensures that the risk assessment remains current and effective in addressing workplace hazards. It allows for the identification of new risks or changes in existing risks, prompting updates to control measures as necessary. While this is important, it should be part of an ongoing process after monitoring the situation rather than the immediate next step after implementing new measures.

Risk assessment is an ongoing process, and assuming that no further action is needed would be incorrect. Even after implementing manual handling aids, continuous monitoring and review are essential to ensure that the measures are effective and that any new risks are promptly addressed. Complacency can lead to overlooked hazards and increased risk of injury, making it crucial to maintain an active approach to risk management.

Source: www.hse.gov.uk/pubns/priced/l23.pdf

QUESTION 42

A 30-year-old laboratory technician has been exposed to a chemical spill in the lab. The spill was quickly contained, but the technician was exposed to a low concentration of the chemical for an extended period before the area was ventilated. You are reviewing the incident to determine the potential health impact of the exposure.

Which of the following best explains how the total dose of chemical exposure is calculated in this scenario?

The answer is: b) Dose = Concentration × Time

Dose calculation: the total dose of a chemical exposure is calculated by multiplying the concentration of the chemical by the duration of exposure (time). This relationship helps assess the potential health impact by considering both how much of the chemical was present and how long the individual was exposed.

Understanding this relationship is crucial for evaluating the severity of exposure incidents.

QUESTION 43

You see Mr Jones, a postal worker who was referred for advice regarding his return to work. Mr Jones tells you that he went off sick after he was bitten by a dog while delivering a parcel. He required antibiotics and stitches but was not admitted to hospital. He has been absent for two weeks to date. His wound is healing well.

Which of the following is the most appropriate advice for you to give the employer regarding the Reporting of Injuries, Diseases and Dangerous Occurrences Regulations 2013 (RIDDOR)?

The answer is: c) This is RIDDOR reportable as he has had more than 7 days of absence due to the incident

The Reporting of Injuries, Diseases and Dangerous Occurrences Regulations 2013 (RIDDOR) require employers and self-employed individuals to report certain workplace incidents.

These include:
- fatalities and specified injuries
- occupational diseases (e.g. carpal tunnel syndrome, dermatitis)
- over-seven-day incapacitation of workers
- injuries to non-workers leading to hospitalisation.

Reports help the HSE monitor and prevent workplace hazards.

RIDDOR covers work-related injuries, not just occupational diseases. While it is true that the incident is not an occupational disease, it is still reportable as a work-related injury.

According to RIDDOR, employers must report work-related accidents that result in an employee being absent from work or unable to perform their normal duties for more than 7 consecutive days (not counting the day of the accident). Since Mr Jones has been absent for 2 weeks due to a work-related injury, this incident is reportable.

As an OH professional, you can provide advice on whether an incident is RIDDOR reportable. However, the responsibility for reporting lies with the employer.

Source: www.hse.gov.uk/riddor/reportable-incidents.htm

QUESTION 44

You are seeing a 34-year-old park ranger to give advice on his return to work. He describes sickness absence due to flu-like illness with a "bull's-eye" rash, which needed treatment with antibiotics.

What is the most likely diagnosis?

The answer is: c) Lyme disease

The patient's symptoms, including the flu-like illness and the characteristic "bull's-eye" rash, along with the need for antibiotic treatment, strongly suggest Lyme disease, particularly given his occupational exposure as a park ranger in an area where ticks are common.

Lyme disease is an infection caused by the *Borrelia burgdorferi* bacteria, transmitted by ticks. It often presents with a characteristic "bull's-eye" rash (erythema migrans) and flu-like symptoms. Treatment involves doxycycline.

Cellulitis is a bacterial infection of the skin and subcutaneous tissues that typically presents with redness, swelling, warmth and pain. It does not typically present with a "bull's-eye" rash or flu-like symptoms prior to the onset of localised symptoms.

Erythema multiforme is an acute, self-limiting skin condition often caused by infections, particularly herpes simplex virus. It presents with target-like lesions but usually involves mucous membranes and widespread lesions. Although it can present with target lesions, these are not typically described as "bull's-eye" and the condition usually involves more widespread lesions and often affects mucous membranes. It is also not commonly treated with antibiotics unless there is an underlying infection requiring such treatment.

Ringworm is a fungal infection of the skin presenting as a red, ring-shaped rash that can be itchy. It is also known as tinea. While ringworm can present with a ring-shaped rash, it is typically not described as a "bull's-eye" rash. It also does not cause flu-like symptoms and is treated with antifungals, not antibiotics.

Source: www.gov.uk/guidance/lyme-disease-differential-diagnosis

QUESTION 45

You receive a query from a new administrator in your occupational health company. She has received a call from a client where you undertake health surveillance for vibration exposure. The administrator informs you that one of the employees has completed their annual questionnaire which indicates that they need further assessment.

Which tier of surveillance for hand arm vibration syndrome (HAVS) is the most appropriate next step?

The answer is: c) Tier 3

This employee has had Tier 2 screening, as indicated by the annual questionnaire. The most appropriate next step is to proceed with Tier 3, which involves a clinical assessment by an OH professional. This step is essential to determine if the employee's symptoms warrant a formal diagnosis or further intervention.

Tier 3 involves a detailed clinical assessment by an OH professional, triggered when the annual screening questionnaire (Tier 2) indicates potential symptoms or issues. This is the appropriate next step given that the employee's questionnaire responses have raised concerns.

Health surveillance tiers for vibration exposure:

Tier 1	Initial assessment	To assess new employees' fitness for work involving vibration exposure via a questionnaire: it focuses on medical history and conditions related to hand or arm disorders and indicates if referral to Tier 3 is needed before the employee starts exposure
Tier 2	Annual screening	To annually monitor employees exposed to vibration risks via an annual questionnaire similar to Tier 1 but issued yearly. If any 'yes' responses are recorded, it triggers a referral to Tier 3 for a detailed clinical assessment
Tier 3	Clinical assessment	To conduct a detailed clinical evaluation by an OH clinician (can be an OH nurse) via a clinical history and examination which focuses on symptoms and clinical signs of potential vibration-related disease
		If vibration-related occupational disease is suspected, advice on fitness for work and potential restriction of vibration exposure is given
		The employee is referred to Tier 4 for formal diagnosis
Tier 4	Diagnosis	To obtain a formal diagnosis by a specialist doctor, usually an OHP; confirms or revises previous advice
		Outcomes can include recommendations on fitness for work and redeployment to roles with no or reduced vibration exposure, or regular reassessments
		Ensures appropriate work assignments and ongoing monitoring of diagnosed employees
Tier 5	Optional testing	Provides additional specialised testing if required or if there is doubt about the diagnosis via a specialist referral to aid a diagnosis

Source: www.hse.gov.uk/pubns/priced/l140.pdf

QUESTION 46

You see a 25-year-old abattoir worker who has been referred by management for advice following his recent diagnosis of attention deficit hyperactivity disorder (ADHD). You notice a lesion on his hand, which he explained started as an "insect bite" and then became a blister. On examination, there is a 3 cm ulcer surrounded by small blisters with marked swelling of the surrounding skin with a central black scab.

What is the most likely diagnosis?

The answer is: a) Anthrax

The description of the lesion is highly characteristic of cutaneous anthrax, which typically starts as a small lesion that develops into a blister and then an ulcer with a central black eschar (scab). The presence of surrounding blisters and significant swelling aligns with cutaneous anthrax symptoms.

The patient is an abattoir worker, which puts him at risk of zoonotic infections, including anthrax. Anthrax is caused by *Bacillus anthracis*, which can be contracted from handling infected animal products.

The differential diagnosis includes:

Lyme disease: this typically presents with erythema migrans, a "bull's-eye" rash, which is not described in this case.

Insect bite: while insect bites can lead to blisters and swelling, they generally do not progress to a necrotic ulcer with a black eschar. The lesion described is more severe and specific than a typical insect bite reaction.

Malignant melanoma: this can present as an ulcerated lesion but typically does not have surrounding blisters and marked swelling. The presence of a black eschar is also not characteristic of melanoma.

Orf: a viral infection from sheep and goats causing pustular lesions, usually on the hands. While abattoir workers could contract orf, the lesion typically does not develop a black eschar, which is more indicative of anthrax.

Sources:
- www.hse.gov.uk/agriculture/assets/docs/anthrax.pdf
- Sadhra, S., Bray, A.J. and Boorman, S. (eds) (2022) *Oxford Handbook of Occupational Health*, 3rd edition

QUESTION 47

You are the occupational health physician (OHP) conducting a health promotion session at a battery production facility. During the session, an employee asks about the link between cadmium exposure and cancer.

Which of the following cancers is associated with cadmium exposure?

The answer is: e) All of the above

Cadmium is classified as a human carcinogen associated with an increased risk of several types of cancer, primarily lung. There is also evidence linking it to cancers of other organs such as the prostate, pancreas, kidney, breast and bladder.

Cadmium has many uses, including in the production of batteries, pigments, metal coatings and plastics.

Source: https://progressreport.cancer.gov/prevention/chemical_exposures/cadmium

QUESTION 48

A 30-year-old female laboratory technician presents to the occupational health clinic with concerns about various hazards in her workplace. She works with chemicals and biological samples, and occasionally handles radiation equipment. Recently, she experienced a minor chemical spill, which led her to reflect on the different hazards she faces daily and their potential risks.

Which one of the following best describes the different categories of hazards she might encounter in her workplace?

The answer is: a) Biological, chemical, ergonomic, physical and psychosocial hazards

There are five main types of hazard:

Biological hazards: these include any biological substances that pose a threat to the health of living organisms, primarily humans. In a laboratory setting, this could be exposure to bacteria, viruses or other pathogens in biological samples.

Answers to Mock exam 1

Chemical hazards: these involve hazardous substances that can cause health issues through inhalation, skin contact or ingestion. The chemical spill she experienced is an example of a chemical hazard.

Ergonomic hazards: these relate to the physical conditions that could cause musculoskeletal injuries. In a laboratory, this might include repetitive strain from pipetting or poor workstation set-up.

Physical hazards: these involve environmental factors that can harm an individual without necessarily touching them, such as radiation, which she occasionally handles.

Psychosocial hazards: these include workplace stress, violence and other social factors that can impact mental health and wellbeing.

Source: www.bohs.org/app/uploads/2024/04/Fl.2-M200-Student-Manual-Feb24.pdf

QUESTION 49

You are being shadowed by a medical student. You see a 60-year-old truck driver with a recent diagnosis of epilepsy is undergoing a fitness to drive medical by the occupational health team. The student wants to understand the regulations set by the Driver and Vehicle Licensing Agency (DVLA) regarding the risk of sudden disabling events.

According to DVLA guidelines, what is the maximum acceptable risk of a sudden disabling event in one year in this driver?

The answer is: d) 2% likelihood of an event

For Group 2 licensing (which includes commercial vehicle drivers such as truck drivers), the DVLA defines the maximum acceptable risk of a sudden disabling event as 2% in one year. This stringent threshold is due to the higher safety standards required for commercial driving.

A 20% likelihood of an event is applicable to Group 1 licensing (i.e. cars and motorcycles), not Group 2 licensing.

Source: www.gov.uk/guidance/general-information-assessing-fitness-to-drive

QUESTION 50

You are advising a 36-year-old employee who is pregnant with twins and has had an uncomplicated pregnancy. She wishes to take a 2-hour flight to attend a work-related conference. She will be 22 weeks pregnant. Her employer is seeking guidance on whether she should go.

Considering the general advice for twin pregnancies, what is the most appropriate recommendation?

The answer is: c) The employee can undertake the flight, but she should consult her healthcare provider for personalised advice

The key focus in assessment of fitness to fly is the health and wellbeing of the mother and the baby. Most airlines do not allow travel after 36 weeks for a single pregnancy and after 32 weeks for multiple pregnancies.

While there are general guidelines regarding travel for twin pregnancies, there is no specific restriction at 22 weeks. However, this advice does not address the importance of the employee consulting with her healthcare provider for personalised advice, as you are relying on the employee's declaration that her pregnancy is uncomplicated.

Source: www.caa.co.uk/passengers-and-public/before-you-fly/am-i-fit-to-fly/guidance-for-health-professionals/pregnancy

QUESTION 51

You are the OHP for a local foundry. You have seen a significant increase in workers experiencing heat stress due to high ambient temperatures and thermal radiation in their workplace. Management seeks the best option to mitigate these health risks. They have provided several solutions that they can feasibly implement.

What is the most appropriate way to reduce the risk of heat stress in these workers?

The answer is: b) Improving air movement

Improving air movement is the most effective control measure among the options provided.

Answers to Mock exam 1

According to the hierarchy of control measures, engineering controls rank higher than administrative controls or PPE. Improving air movement falls under engineering controls, which aim to eliminate or minimise the hazard at its source.

Administrative controls: rest breaks are an administrative control that allows workers to recuperate in cooler areas but does not address the root cause of heat stress.

While beneficial, acclimatisation is a gradual process and may not provide immediate relief from current heat stress conditions.

Providing cool water helps with hydration but does not address the thermal environment directly; it is more of a supportive measure alongside primary controls.

QUESTION 52

You are undertaking a workplace visit at a workplace involving welding. One of your students notices a sign on the local exhaust ventilation which states that the last inspection was 12 months ago. The manager assures you that the equipment is in a good state of repair.

When should the business schedule the next inspection?

The answer is: a) 2 months

Local exhaust ventilation can be an important engineering control for airborne hazards. The Control of Substances Hazardous to Health Regulations (COSHH) require the maintenance and thorough examination and testing of control measures at specific intervals to ensure the control measures are effective at all times. The maximum time between tests of local exhaust ventilation systems is set out in COSHH and for most systems this is 14 months.

Source: www.hse.gov.uk/pubns/priced/hsg258.pdf

QUESTION 53

You advise a company on their health surveillance for noise. An employee is moving into a role located within a hearing protection zone. The company wants to know when he should commence participation in the health surveillance programme.

What is the most appropriate response?

The answer is: e) It is appropriate to have a health surveillance review prior to starting in the new job role

Health surveillance should be targeted based on the actual exposure risk to noise. If the employee was not previously working in a hearing protection zone, there may not have been a need for health surveillance until now.

If he is working in a designated hearing protection zone this implies that the upper limit value is exceeded for noise exposure and therefore there is a requirement for health surveillance.

Ideally, health surveillance should commence before individuals are exposed to noise, such as for new employees or those changing job roles, to establish a baseline hearing status before exposure to noise requiring hearing protection begins. This allows for effective monitoring of any changes in hearing health over time.

However, it can be implemented at any time for employees already exposed to noise. This is followed by a series of regular checks, typically annually for the first two years of employment, and then at three-year intervals thereafter. The frequency may need to increase if hearing problems are detected or if the risk of hearing damage remains high.

Source: www.hse.gov.uk/noise/healthsurveillance.htm

QUESTION 54

You are asked to give an opinion on fitness to work for a veterinary surgeon who is 15 weeks pregnant. It is birthing season at the farm where she works. She is worried about exposure to *Coxiella burnetii*.

What is the most appropriate opinion to give?

The answer is: b) She needs to be removed from delivering calves and lambs

Q fever is caused by the *Coxiella burnetii* organism, and is widespread globally among livestock and domestic ruminants. Sheep, cattle and goats are the most frequent source of human infection.

Infection in pregnant women can have an adverse effect on the developing foetus, including premature birth or abortion and low birth weight. Pregnant women are therefore advised to avoid contact with these pregnant animals.

To avoid the possible risk of infection, pregnant women should not help ewes to lamb, nor provide assistance with a cow that is calving or a nanny goat that is kidding. They should avoid contact with aborted or newborn lambs, calves or kids or with the afterbirth, birthing fluids or materials (e.g. bedding or clothing) contaminated by such birth products, vaccines or recently vaccinated sheep and material that may have come into contact with the above.

Sources:
- https://phw.nhs.wales/news/advice-issued-to-pregnant-women-during-lambing-season/#:~:text=To%20avoid%20the%20possible%20risk,birthing%20fluids%20or%20materials%20
- www.gov.uk/guidance/q-fever

QUESTION 55

You are an OH professional evaluating an office environment where several employees have reported symptoms such as headaches, dizziness and eye irritation. Some of the staff believe these symptoms are caused by the building environment, and there is concern that this might indicate a serious workplace illness.

Which of the following statements best describes 'sick building syndrome'?

The answer is: c) Sick building syndrome refers to a set of symptoms reported by building occupants that cannot be traced to a specific illness or hazard

Sick building syndrome is a term used to describe a collection of non-specific symptoms – such as headaches, dizziness and eye irritation – that some building occupants experience without a clearly identifiable cause.

Source: www.hse.gov.uk/pubns/priced/hsg132.pdf

QUESTION 56

You see a 52-year-old office worker who has been referred one week after a transient ischaemic attack (TIA) for advice on return to work. He is eager to return to his routine, and commutes for one hour each day by car for employment.

What is the most appropriate advice regarding his return to driving?

The answer is: b) He must not drive for 1 month after a TIA and does not need to notify the DVLA

For Group 1 drivers (car and motorcycle), individuals must not drive for 1 month after a TIA but do not need to notify the DVLA. If more than one TIA occurs, a one-month driving restriction is required after each episode.

For Group 2 drivers (bus and lorry), they must not drive and must notify the DVLA. Their licence will be revoked for one year following a stroke or TIA. Relicensing after one year is possible if there is no residual impairment affecting safe driving and no significant risk factor, and may be subject to a satisfactory medical report.

Source: https://assets.publishing.service.gov.uk/media/65cf7243e1bdec001a322268/assessing-fitness-to-drive-february-2024.pdf

QUESTION 57

A 50-year-old employee has recently been evaluated by you for a work-related health issue, and a report has been prepared for their employer stating that the patient is fit for work. The employee now wishes to withdraw consent for the report to be disclosed to their employer, expressing disagreement with your opinion that they are fit to work.

What is the most appropriate course of action if an employee withdraws consent for the disclosure of a report?

The answer is: b) Notify the report commissioner of the employee's withdrawal of consent, but withhold the report and do not disclose any further information

Option b) adheres to the principles of confidentiality and patient autonomy. If a patient withdraws consent, you must inform the report commissioner of the withdrawal but respect the patient's wishes by not disclosing the report to the employer. Disclosure of the report without consent is not appropriate unless legally required or justified in the public interest.

Source: www.fom.ac.uk/wp-content/uploads/GOMP_2017_Web.pdf

QUESTION 58

You are working with the safety team, evaluating a risk assessment of a workplace using toluene.

The workers are using respiratory protection equipment (RPE) with an assigned protection factor (APF) of 200.

The measured airborne toluene concentration: 500 ppm (parts per million) within an 8-hour time-weighted average (TWA).

Toluene WEL (workplace exposure limit): 50 ppm (from EH40).

What is the lowest assigned protection factor that should be used for the employee's respiratory protection equipment?

The answer is: c) 20

The EH40 is the Health and Safety Executive (HSE) official reference document on WELs to be used alongside the Control of Substances Hazardous to Health (COSHH) Regulations 2002. The document guides those responsible for controlling exposure to hazardous substances at work.

Measured airborne toluene concentration: 500 ppm (parts per million) within an 8-hour TWA.

Toluene WEL: 50 ppm (from EH40).

Required APF to reduce to WEL = 500/50 = 10.

When calculating the protection factor, always choose an APF above the calculated value. In this case an APF of 20 is the minimum protection required.

RPE type and class is categorised by an assigned protection factor (APF). The APF is a number rating that indicates how much protection that RPE is capable of providing. For example, RPE with an APF of 10 will reduce the wearer's exposure by at least a factor of 10 if used properly, or, to put it another way, the wearer will only breathe in one-tenth or less of the amount of substance present in the air.

There are only a few number ratings used, so RPE APFs will be one of: 4; 10; 20; 40; 200; or 2000.

Source: www.hse.gov.uk/pubns/guidance/rseries.htm

QUESTION 59

You are the OHP reviewing the health questionnaire of a pregnant nurse prior to starting work on the renal ward. She has no history of chickenpox or shingles, nor vaccination / passive immunity against VZV.

What is the most appropriate next step in managing this pregnant healthcare worker's potential exposure to VZV (varicella zoster virus)?

The answer is: d) Test her for VZV antibodies

Pregnant healthcare workers without a history of chickenpox or shingles should be tested for VZV antibodies to determine their immunity status. If they are found to be antibody negative, VZV immunoglobulin should be administered to provide passive immunity and reduce the risk of varicella, which can be more severe during pregnancy.

While avoiding exposure to VZV is important, this option does not address the immediate need to test her immunity and provide VZIG if necessary.

Sources:
- www.nhshealthatwork.co.uk/images/library/files/Clinical%20excellence/Varicella_zoster_guidelines_web_navigable.pdf
- https://assets.publishing.service.gov.uk/media/66faaaf2a31f45a9c765eeb1/Green-book-Chapter-34-Varicella_25_9_24.pdf

QUESTION 60

A health and safety officer is conducting a health promotion seminar for office workers who use display screen equipment (DSE). During the seminar, one of the employees asks about the most common health problems associated with DSE work.

Which of the following health problems is related to DSE work?

The answer is: d) Upper limb disorders

The main hazards associated with DSE work encompass musculoskeletal disorders, fatigue and stress, and eye and eyesight effects.

Musculoskeletal disorders (MSDs): MSDs affecting the upper limbs (ULDs/WRULDs) are prevalent among DSE users. These disorders range from temporary fatigue or soreness to chronic conditions such as carpal tunnel syndrome. Factors contributing to MSDs include poor workstation ergonomics, prolonged static postures and repetitive tasks. Psychosocial factors such as high workloads and tight deadlines also play a significant role in the onset of MSDs.

Fatigue and stress: prolonged or intense periods of stress are common among DSE workers, and can lead to physical and mental health issues. Stress can exacerbate symptoms related to upper limb and visual problems. Psychosocial risk factors include lack of control over work methods, high attention demands and insufficient social interaction.

Eye and eyesight effects: DSE work does not cause permanent eye damage, but it can lead to temporary visual symptoms such as blurred vision, eye strain and headaches. Poor workstation set-up, including inadequate lighting or screen glare, contributes to visual discomfort. Pre-existing vision defects may become more noticeable, increasing the risk of musculoskeletal disorders due to altered posture.

Source: www.hse.gov.uk/pubns/priced/l26.pdf

QUESTION 61

You are working as a contractor at a car manufacturing site. The employer wants you to help assess the ergonomic risks on the assembly line.

What is the most appropriate tool to use?

The answer is: a) ART tool

The Assessment of Repetitive Tasks (ART) tool is specifically designed to assess ergonomic risks associated with repetitive tasks involving the upper limbs, which are common on an assembly line in a car manufacturing site. This tool helps identify risks related to repetitive motion, force, awkward postures and duration of tasks, making it the most appropriate for assessing the ergonomic risks on an assembly line.

The Risk Assessment of Pushing and Pulling (RAPP) tool is designed to assess the risks associated with manual handling tasks that involve pushing and pulling. While useful in contexts where such activities are prevalent, it is less relevant to an assembly line, where repetitive tasks involving the upper limbs are more common. Therefore, it is not the most appropriate tool for this scenario.

The Manual Handling Assessment Charts (MAC) tool is used to assess the risk of injury from manual handling activities such as lifting, carrying and team handling. While some manual handling may occur on an assembly line, the primary focus is on repetitive tasks involving the upper limbs, making the ART tool more suitable than the MAC tool for this specific assessment.

The QRISK tool is a general risk assessment tool used to evaluate cardiovascular risk factors, typically in a healthcare setting. It is not designed for assessing ergonomic risks in a workplace environment, particularly not for an assembly line in a car manufacturing site. Therefore, this tool is not relevant to the scenario and is the least appropriate option.

The V-MAC tool is a variation of the MAC tool, focusing on more specific aspects of manual handling. Similarly to the MAC tool, it does not comprehensively address the repetitive tasks involving the upper limbs that are prevalent on an assembly line. Hence, it is less appropriate than the ART tool for this particular assessment.

Source: www.hse.gov.uk/msd/uld/art/resources.htm

QUESTION 62

A 45-year-old male construction worker visits the clinic for health surveillance. During the examination, he expresses concerns about his workplace, specifically about the potential for asbestos exposure. He has read that asbestos is dangerous and is worried about the implications for his health.

What is the most appropriate way to explain the difference between hazard and risk in the context of his concern about asbestos exposure?

The answer is: a) Hazard refers to the inherent potential of asbestos to cause harm, whereas risk is the likelihood that this harm will occur given the level of exposure

Hazard is the potential to cause harm or adverse effect. For example, mesothelioma may arise from exposure to the hazard of asbestos.

Risk is the probability that a hazard will be realised, given the nature and extent of a person's exposure to an agent or circumstance. For example, the risk of mesothelioma from asbestos depends on the type of fibre and the amount that is inhaled.

Sources:
- www.hsa.ie/eng/topics/hazards
- Sadhra, S., Bray, A.J. and Boorman, S. (eds) (2022) *Oxford Handbook of Occupational Health*, 3rd edition

QUESTION 63

You are an OHP assessing a 60-year-old ex-construction worker who has recently been diagnosed with lung cancer, believed to be related to prolonged asbestos exposure. The worker is seeking advice on their eligibility for the Industrial Injuries Disablement Benefit (IIDB) and wants to understand the criteria for receiving this benefit.

To qualify for the IIDB, what is the minimum level of disability (expressed as a percentage) that this worker needs to be assessed as having?

The answer is: b) The worker must be assessed as at least 14% disabled

The amount of benefit a person may receive is determined by the level of their disability, which is assessed by a 'medical advisor' on a scale of 1 to 100%.

Generally, an individual must be assessed as being 14% disabled or more to qualify for the benefit. The exception is noise-induced hearing loss, where the level of disability must be assessed as over 20%.

Sources:
- www.gov.uk/industrial-injuries-disablement-benefit/what-youll-get
- Sadhra, S., Bray, A.J. and Boorman, S. (eds) (2022) *Oxford Handbook of Occupational Health*, 3rd edition

QUESTION 64

You are teaching a group of occupational medicine trainees about the adverse health effects of noise exposure. One student has a query about noise-induced hearing loss:

Which one of the following types of pathology is noise-induced hearing loss?

The answer is: b) Sensorineural hearing loss

Noise-induced hearing loss is sensorineural hearing loss, affecting the cochlear hair cells in the inner ear due to prolonged or excessive exposure to loud noise.

Source: www.som.org.uk/sites/som.org.uk/files/SOM_UKHCA_Position_Statement_Noise_Health_Surveillance_Guidance_May_23.pdf

QUESTION 65

You see a 30-year-old baker with a 6-month history of erythema and vesicles on his hands. On examination, there are multiple vesicles and erythematous skin patches, along with some areas of lichenification. There is no evidence of wheals. He describes a pattern of skin disease that worsens at work and improves during holidays. He has no relevant past medical history.

What would be the most appropriate next step in the investigation?

The answer is: b) Patch test

This employee's history and examination findings are consistent with occupational allergic dermatitis.

Common sensitisers include soaps, nickel (cheap jewellery) and rubber.

If allergic dermatitis is suspected, patch testing may be performed. This test involves applying various test substances to the skin under adhesive tape, which are then left in place for 48 hours. The skin is examined upon removal of these patches and again 48 hours later for any response.

This can help identify which allergens the employee may be allergic to, and which ones might be aggravating the dermatitis.

Patch testing is typically carried out by a dermatologist.

The other investigations are not appropriate to make this diagnosis.

Answers to Mock exam 1

Sources:
- www.hsa.ie/eng/workplace_health/occupational_asthma_and_dermatitis/occupational_dermatitis_frequently_asked_questions/#:~:text=The%20assessment%20may%20include%20an,in%20place%20for%2048%20hours
- Sadhra, S., Bray, A.J. and Boorman, S. (eds) (2022) *Oxford Handbook of Occupational Health*, 3rd edition

QUESTION 66

A 45-year-old site manager at a construction company is responsible for ensuring the safety of the workers on site. During a safety meeting, a new regulation is discussed, which requires the manager to formally identify and evaluate potential hazards that could harm the workers. The manager is unsure which specific legislation mandates this requirement for a risk assessment.

Which legislation introduced the concept of mandatory risk assessment in the workplace?

The answer is: b) The Management of Health and Safety at Work Regulations 1999

The Management of Health and Safety at Work Regulations 1999: these regulations specifically introduce the requirement for employers to carry out risk assessments to identify and evaluate risks to health and safety. They mandate the systematic approach to hazard identification and risk control in the workplace.

The Health and Safety at Work Act 1974: this provides a general framework for workplace health and safety but does not specifically mandate risk assessments.

The Control of Substances Hazardous to Health Regulations 2002: while these regulations require risk assessments for hazardous substances, they do not introduce the general concept of risk assessment for all workplace hazards.

The Personal Protective Equipment at Work Regulations 1992: these regulations require employers to provide PPE where risks cannot be adequately controlled by other means, but they do not introduce the concept of risk assessment.

The Workplace (Health, Safety and Welfare) Regulations 1992: these regulations set out the basic requirements for the workplace environment, but do not introduce the concept of risk assessment.

Source: www.hse.gov.uk/pubns/hsc13.pdf

QUESTION 67

You are advising a private health clinic that is moving from lower level skin surveillance to a higher level skin surveillance programme following a new case of occupational dermatitis in the workplace.

What is the most appropriate step to be added to the previous health surveillance programme?

The answer is: e) Regular visual skin inspections by a responsible persons

Suitable health surveillance for occupational contact dermatitis involves different levels of monitoring based on the risk and exposure factors.

Higher level health surveillance

Appropriate when: there is clear evidence of a hazard or potential for significant exposure to substances or processes known to cause occupational contact dermatitis. This includes industries where dermatitis is common despite risk reduction measures.

Actions include:
- assessing workers' skin condition before or soon after starting a relevant job, to establish a baseline
- regular visual skin inspections by a responsible person, typically on a brief monthly routine
- educating employees about likely exposures and symptoms to watch for
- instructing employees on how and to whom to report symptoms occurring between inspections
- a prescribed schedule of employee questionnaires for additional feedback and monitoring.

Lower level health surveillance

Appropriate when: exposure is occasional, controls are adequate, or based on consultation with a health professional.

Actions include:
- conducting an annual questionnaire administered by a trained responsible person
- informing employees about potential exposures and symptoms to monitor
- Instructing employees on reporting procedures for symptoms if they arise.

Overall, the level of health surveillance for occupational contact dermatitis should align with the level of risk and exposure in the workplace. Higher levels of surveillance are warranted where there is significant exposure or a known risk, while lower levels may suffice when exposure and risk are minimal and controlled. Regular education, monitoring and reporting mechanisms are essential components of both levels of surveillance to ensure early detection and effective management of dermatitis risks among workers.

Source: www.som.org.uk/sites/som.org.uk/files/SOM_Managing_Skin_Health_at_Work_Nov_2023.pdf

QUESTION 68

You are an OH professional reviewing the health surveillance protocols for a company where employees are exposed to whole body vibration (WBV) due to the use of heavy machinery. The company wants to ensure compliance with current regulations and best practices.

Which of the following statements is true regarding health surveillance for employees exposed to whole body vibration?

The answer is: b) Health surveillance is not appropriate for WBV

Routine health surveillance is not appropriate for WBV. This is confirmed as the HSE position in which it states that "health surveillance is not appropriate for WBV because it is considered that no methods currently exist for detecting changes in people's backs, which can reliably indicate the early onset of changes (which may cause low back pain) that are specifically related to workplace factors". The HSE suggests that 'health monitoring' may be helpful, but this is not a legal requirement under the Control of Vibrations at Work Regulations 2005, and reflects a holistic approach to back pain, using an annual checklist for employees at risk.

Source: www.som.org.uk/sites/som.org.uk/files/HAVS_and_Whole_Body_Vibration_Feb_2023.pdf

QUESTION 69

You are a newly qualified OHP and have been asked to conduct a medical examination for a group of workers who are exposed to hazardous substances. Your supervisor informs you that the examination must be conducted by an 'appointed doctor' according to statutory requirements.

Which of the following best describes the primary role of an 'appointed doctor'?

The answer is: c) To conduct statutory medical surveillance

An 'appointed doctor' is a registered medical practitioner designated by the HSE to perform statutory medical surveillance for workers exposed to specific hazards. Their role is to ensure that occupational health standards are maintained and that workers are fit to work in environments where they may be exposed to hazardous substances. This role is different from general medical care, routine health checks or counselling, which are not statutory requirements under OH regulations.

QUESTION 70

A construction worker presents with symptoms of carpal tunnel syndrome (CTS). He reports using vibratory tools frequently in his job. A vibration risk assessment performed since his symptoms started shows vibration exposure is kept as low as reasonably practicable.

What is the most appropriate recommendation for his employer to reduce his risk of worsening CTS?

The answer is: c) Advise the employer to conduct an ergonomic assessment

Since a vibration risk assessment has already been performed and exposure is minimised, the next best step is for the employer to perform an ergonomic assessment. This will help identify and modify tasks that involve repetitive or forceful wrist movements, especially those performed in non-neutral positions. Addressing ergonomic factors can significantly reduce strain on the wrists and help prevent further aggravation of CTS symptoms.

Source: www.som.org.uk/sites/som.org.uk/files/Carpal_tunnel_syndrome_and_work_with_hand-held_vibrating_tools_Jan2022.pdf

Answers to Mock exam 1

QUESTION 71

You are a new OHP. You see Mr McDougall, who has given consent for their report to be released, and stated that they do not wish to see their report prior to its dissemination.

What is the recommended best practice in this situation?

The answer is: c) Send a copy of the report to the worker at the same time as you send it to the referrer

Sending a copy of the report to the worker at the same time as you send it to the referrer ensures transparency, maintains trust, and allows the worker to access the report directly if they choose to do so later.

Source: Faculty of Occupational Medicine (2018) *Ethics Guidance for Occupational Health Practice*, 8th edition

QUESTION 72

You are discussing the role of the Employment Medical Advisory Service (EMAS) with a group of occupational medicine trainees.

Which one of the following is a responsibility of EMAS staff?

The answer is: e) Investigate ill-health reports received under the Reporting of Injuries, Diseases and Dangerous Occurrences Regulations 2013 (RIDDOR)

EMAS provides expert, independent services by:
- investigating health complaints from employers, employees, unions and the public
- reviewing ill-health reports under RIDDOR (2013)
- assisting HSE inspectors and local authorities to ensure compliance with health and safety laws
- offering workplace advice to employers, employees and trade unions
- providing expert advice to general and OH professionals
- supporting HSE's OH campaigns.

EMAS does not:
- provide medical treatment (they advise family doctors and hospitals)
- offer OH services to organisations (they refer to local services)
- handle nuisance complaints (these go to local authorities)

- provide rehabilitation for disabilities
- conduct most statutory medical exams (these are done by appointed doctors)
- assess first aid training organisations.

Source: www.poauk.org.uk/media/1467/employment-advisory-service-and-you.pdf

QUESTION 73

You see a 60-year-old employee for long-term sickness absence. He tells you he does not want to return to work and has handed in his notice. He asks you how long his occupational health notes and report will be retained by the department. Reports in the department are retained in compliance with General Data Protection Regulations (GDPR).

What is the most appropriate retention period for his occupational health reports?

The answer is: b) His employment period plus 6 years

According to current guidelines, OH reports should be retained for the duration of the person's employment plus 6 years or until their 75th birthday, whichever occurs sooner. This approach ensures compliance with GDPR's storage limitation principle, safeguarding personal data while allowing for necessary retention in case of legal obligations or claims. OH departments should adhere to this guideline to ensure compliance and protect individuals' privacy rights by appropriately managing the retention of occupational health reports.

Source: www.fom.ac.uk/media-events/news/guidance/guidance-on-the-general-data-protection-regulation

QUESTION 74

A 30-year-old healthcare worker has their blood tested for hepatitis B immunity status. Their results are as follows:

HBsAg (hepatitis B surface antigen): Negative

HBsAb (hepatitis B surface antibody): Positive

HBcAb (hepatitis B core antibody): Positive

Answers to Mock exam 1

How best should these results be interpreted, and what action is needed?

The answer is: c) The individual has recovered from a past hepatitis B infection and is protected; no vaccine is needed

The HBsAg test, which indicates an active infection, is negative.

The positive HBsAb indicates protection, and the positive HBcAb suggests that the immunity is from a past infection.

The negative HBsAg indicates that the person is not a carrier.

Source: www.hepb.org/prevention-and-diagnosis/diagnosis/understanding-your-test-results

QUESTION 75

A 45-year-old office worker is recovering from long Covid and is preparing to return to work. The company's policy allows for a phased return to work (RTW) with a maximum duration of 4 weeks.

What is the most appropriate advice for managing RTW in employees recovering from long Covid?

The answer is: b) Individuals recovering from long Covid generally need a longer phased RTW period than the standard 4 weeks

Long Covid can cause prolonged symptoms that often necessitate a more gradual and extended return to work than the standard 4-week policy allows.

Source: www.som.org.uk/sites/som.org.uk/files/SOM_Long_COVID_A_Managers_Guide_April_2024.pdf

QUESTION 76

You are an OH professional reviewing a risk assessment at a bottling factory. You note that static monitoring has shown high noise levels in certain areas. Workers move through various roles throughout their shifts, including assembly lines.

Which of the following is the most appropriate method for accurately measuring an employee's exposure to noise over a work shift?

The answer is: b) Dosimeter

89

A dosimeter is a personal sound level meter, specifically designed to measure an individual's cumulative noise exposure over time, and therefore is the most appropriate answer. Since workers in the bottling factory move between different areas and roles, a dosimeter, which can be worn on the person, provides an accurate measurement of the varying noise levels the employee is exposed to throughout their shift without interrupting their work.

A sound level meter also measures noise levels and can be a hand-held portable instrument. To take measurements, the sound level meter (SLM) is held at arm's length at the ear height for those exposed to the noise.

A photometer measures light intensity and is not relevant for noise exposure assessment.

A personal noise alarm alerts workers when noise levels exceed a certain threshold, but does not measure or log noise exposure over time.

An accelerometer measures vibration and movement, not noise levels. It is not applicable for measuring noise exposure in this context.

Source: Sadhra, S., Bray, A.J. and Boorman, S. (eds) (2022) *Oxford Handbook of Occupational Health*, 3rd edition

QUESTION 77

You are teaching a group of diploma students about the effects of radiation in the workplace. One student asks you what the 'effective dose' means.

What is the most appropriate answer?

The answer is: c) Takes into account the concentration of energy deposited in tissue as a result of an exposure to ionising radiation, the relative harm level of the radiation, and the sensitivities of each organ to radiation

Absorbed dose: this is the measure of energy deposition in any irradiated material by all types of ionising radiation.

Equivalent dose: in biological systems, the same absorbed dose of different types of radiation produces different degrees of biological damage. This measurement takes into account the damaging properties of different radiation types and therefore describes the impact of radiation type on tissue.

Effective dose: the risk to various tissues varies from one tissue to another; it is not the same for any given equivalent dose. The effective dose is the calculated value considering:
- absorbed dose to all body organs
- relative harm level of the radiation
- sensitivities of each organ to radiation.

It is a single measure of the risk of detriment to health.

Sources:
- www.radiologyinfo.org/en/info/safety-hiw_09
- Sadhra, S., Bray, A.J. and Boorman, S. (eds) (2022) *Oxford Handbook of Occupational Health*, 3rd edition

QUESTION 78

Which one of the following regulations is not part of the 'Six Pack' regulations in the UK?

The answer is: b) Reporting of Injuries, Diseases and Dangerous Occurrences Regulations 2013

The 'Six Pack' regulations are a set of UK health and safety regulations designed to ensure compliance with the Health and Safety at Work Act 1974. They comprise the following:
1. Management of Health and Safety at Work Regulations 1999: focus on risk assessments and health and safety management.
2. Personal Protective Equipment Regulations 2002: govern the use of personal protective equipment at work.
3. Workplace (Health, Safety and Welfare) Regulations 1992: cover basic health, safety and welfare requirements.
4. The Provision and Use of Work Equipment Regulations 1998: relate to the safe use of equipment.
5. Health and Safety (Display Screen Equipment) Regulations 1992: provide guidelines for working with display screen equipment.
6. Manual Handling Operations Regulations 1992: focus on the safe handling of loads.

Reporting of Injuries, Diseases and Dangerous Occurrences Regulations (RIDDOR) 2013 is not part of the 'Six Pack' regulations. It focuses on the reporting of work-related accidents, diseases and dangerous occurrences.

QUESTION 79

A 50-year-old man undergoes a routine hearing test as part of his OH surveillance. The audiogram shows that the difference of the sum of the hearing levels at 1, 2, 3 and 4 kHz for both ears is greater than 40 dB.

What is the most appropriate next step in management?

The answer is: c) Refer back to GP/ENT to exclude acoustic neuroma

Significant unilateral hearing loss should prompt further investigation to exclude serious causes such as an acoustic neuroma. This requires referral to an ear, nose and throat (ENT) specialist (normally via the GP) for assessment and likely an MRI scan. While noise-induced hearing loss is common, asymmetry in hearing loss should raise concern for other underlying pathologies, making option c) the most appropriate next step.

Sources:
- www.som.org.uk/sites/som.org.uk/files/Supplementary_Guidance_on_Interpreting_an_Audiogram_for_Indications_of_Occupational_NIHL_Sept_2024.pdf
- Sadhra, S., Bray, A.J. and Boorman, S. (eds) (2022) *Oxford Handbook of Occupational Health*, 3rd edition

QUESTION 80

Which of the following statements most accurately reflects the challenges faced by younger workers during and after the Covid-19 pandemic, compared to older workers?

The answer is: b) Younger workers are more likely to exhibit presenteeism

The concept of presenteeism is becoming increasingly significant in the workplace. It refers to employees attending work while unwell, which impairs their ability to perform effectively. Additionally, younger individuals, especially those on precarious contracts, are more likely to work while sick due to job insecurity and therefore are more likely to exhibit presenteeism.

Younger workers, especially those aged 16–24, have been disproportionately affected by recent economic challenges and were more likely to be furloughed during the pandemic.

Older workers are more at risk of long-term unemployment. The number of unemployed over-50s has increased well above other age groups.

Reluctance to report mental health problems is common among younger workers, who are less likely to disclose such issues to employers.

Many younger workers are employed in sectors that have been severely affected by the Covid-19 pandemic, such as retail and hospitality. Workers under the age of 25 are approximately 2.5 times more likely to be in these vulnerable sectors compared to older age groups, and therefore are more likely to work in sectors affected by the Covid-19 pandemic. Young women, in particular, are notably represented in these at-risk industries.

Sources:
- https://www.som.org.uk/Supporting_businesses_to_build_back_better_The_benefits_of_age_diversity.pdf
- https://oshwiki.osha.europa.eu/en/themes/presenteeism-overview

QUESTIONS for Mock exam 2

QUESTION 1

A study is investigating the link between substance Y and lung cancer. Researchers find that individuals who worked in industries linked to substance Y exposure had a higher incidence of lung cancer. They want to use the Bradford Hill criteria to demonstrate an association.

Which of the following best defines the Bradford Hill criterion of temporality in this context?

a) The exposure and the disease must be consistently linked across different studies and populations
b) A demonstration that the cause precedes the effect
c) The strength of the association between the exposure and the disease must be strong
d) Higher exposure levels lead to a higher risk of the disease
e) Similar exposures in other contexts or conditions should lead to similar diseases

QUESTION 2

You are conducting a workplace health and safety review for a large retailer. The employer is concerned about the risk of Covid-19 among employees and wants to identify individuals who may be more susceptible to severe outcomes if they contract the virus. You are asked to provide guidance on the factors that increase individual susceptibility to severe Covid-19 infection.

Which of the following is a factor that most increases individual susceptibility to severe Covid-19 infection?

a) Immunosuppressive treatment
b) Black and Asian ethnicity

c) Obesity
d) Pregnancy
e) All of the above

QUESTION 3

You are consulted to provide guidance on which types of procedures pose a risk of transmitting blood-borne viruses (BBVs) from the healthcare worker (HCW) to the patient.

Which of the following best describes an exposure-prone procedure (EPP)?

a) Any procedure where the HCW's hands are always visible
b) Procedures where the HCW's blood may contaminate the patient's open tissues if an injury occurs
c) Any procedure involving HCW contact with a patient's mucous membranes
d) Procedures where the HCW is at high risk of needlestick injuries
e) Procedures where the HCW is required to wear personal protective equipment (PPE)

QUESTION 4

You are teaching occupational medicine trainees about identifying factors that could influence an individual's susceptibility to prolonged illness or sickness absence.

In the context of the flags system used for this purpose, which of the following is most appropriately considered a 'chequered flag'?

a) Beliefs about pain and injury that are potentially changeable during consultations
b) Company policies affecting financial security and communication issues with the employer
c) Low job satisfaction and excessive work demands that may be modifiable with early intervention
d) Psychological distress and unhelpful coping strategies that could be addressed through behaviour change methods
e) Social factors such as caregiving responsibilities or other commitments outside of work

QUESTION 5

You are working for a large office-based company with 10 000 employees. As a result of the Covid-19 pandemic, its employees are now all agile workers. The company wants to know how to fulfil its health and safety duties to employees working from home.

What is the most appropriate advice to give the employer?

a) Employees should check with their home insurer and their mortgage provider or landlord that they can work from home
b) No action needs to be taken – it is the employee's duty to ensure that they are safe when working from home
c) The employer should make sure their insurance covers employees working from home
d) The employer should provide their employees with information to do a self-risk assessment of their home
e) The employer should undertake a home visit to perform a risk assessment to ensure the working environment is safe

QUESTION 6

During an annual review of anonymised health surveillance audiometric results, it is observed that there has been a deterioration in hearing among a specific group of workers.

What is the most appropriate next step in response to these findings?

a) Continue with the current noise control measures and monitor hearing levels intensively over the next year
b) Reassess the exposure factors to identify potential changes in exposure conditions that may have contributed to the deterioration
c) Reassess these workers as soon as feasible
d) Recommend that all workers immediately increase their use of hearing protection
e) Provide additional training to employees on the importance of hearing conservation methods

QUESTION 7

You are an occupational health and safety officer conducting a routine inspection at a manufacturing plant. During your visit, an employee mentions that they want to sign a disclaimer to opt out of wearing the required personal protective equipment (PPE) because they find it uncomfortable and believe the risk in their specific role is minimal. The employee asks if this is permissible.

What is the most appropriate response to the employee's request to sign a disclaimer to not wear PPE?

a) Allow the employee to sign a disclaimer as long as they accept full responsibility for any injuries sustained
b) Allow the employee to sign a disclaimer after providing them with detailed information on the risks and limitations of not wearing PPE
c) Allow the employee to stop wearing PPE if they undertake increased appointments with their GP
d) Inform the employee that signing a disclaimer is not possible, as employers are legally required to provide PPE and ensure its use when risks cannot be controlled in other ways
e) Permit the employee to opt out of wearing PPE for tasks that are low risk, as long as they remain cautious

QUESTION 8

You see an employee who has recently been diagnosed with occupational asthma by a respiratory physician. You are aware that this is a RIDDOR reportable disease.

Which of the following is required to submit reports of injuries, diseases and dangerous occurrences under RIDDOR?

a) The employee
b) The occupational physician
c) The responsible person
d) The manager of the employee
e) All of the above

QUESTION 9

You are an occupational health professional asked to review a group of office workers who have reported a variety of symptoms, including dry or itchy skin, dry or itchy eyes, nose or throat, headaches, lethargy and a runny nose. On examination, all individuals show normal physical findings. Recent inspections of the air conditioning and ventilation systems in the office building were unremarkable.

What is the most likely diagnosis for these workers?

a) Humidifier fever
b) Common cold
c) Sick building syndrome
d) Occupational asthma
e) Legionnaires' disease

QUESTION 10

You are conducting a consultation with an employee, and at the end of the session, they request a copy of their medical records. They ask how long it will take for them to receive this information once they make a formal request.

How long does an organisation have to provide the requested information after a formal Subject Access Request (SAR) is made?

a) 5 working days
b) 2 weeks
c) 1 month
d) 6 weeks
e) 6 months

QUESTION 11

You are working with a manufacturer on their preventive health strategy. You note that a third of their workforce are welders.

Which vaccination is most appropriate to offer this workforce?

a) Covid-19
b) Hepatitis B

c) Influenza
d) Pneumococcal
e) Varicella zoster

QUESTION 12

You are an OHP working in a manufacturing plant where employees are exposed to various hazardous materials. Your employer has asked you to review the need for statutory medical surveillance to ensure compliance with health and safety regulations. You note that the plant uses materials that involve exposure to lead, asbestos and ionising radiation.

Which one professional is specifically appointed by the Health and Safety Executive (HSE) to conduct statutory medical surveillance under specific regulations?

a) Occupational Health Nurse
b) Appointed Doctor
c) Consultant (Accredited Specialist) in Occupational Medicine
d) Occupational Hygienist
e) Health and Safety Officer

QUESTION 13

An employer is reviewing their health and safety protocols for employees who work with ionising radiation.

Under radiation protection regulations, how are employees designated as 'classified persons' when working with ionising radiation?

a) Employees are designated as classified persons if they are likely to receive a personal radiation dose exceeding 1 mSv per year
b) Employees are designated as classified persons if they are likely to receive a personal radiation dose exceeding 3 mSv per year
c) Employees are designated as classified persons if they are likely to receive a personal radiation dose exceeding 6 mSv per year
d) Employees are designated as classified persons if they are likely to receive a personal radiation dose exceeding 10 mSv per year
e) Employees are designated as classified persons based solely on their job role, regardless of the personal radiation dose received

Questions for Mock exam 2

QUESTION 14

You are an occupational health (OH) professional asked to assess an employee who has been off sick for a prolonged period. The manager seeks your opinion on whether the employee should be dismissed due to their inability to work.

What is the most appropriate role of the OH professional in this situation?

a) The OH professional should decide whether the employee should be dismissed based on their medical condition and likelihood of recovery
b) The OH professional should recommend dismissal if the employee is unlikely to return to work within the next 6 months
c) The OH professional should provide and interpret medical information, allowing the employer to make an informed decision about dismissal
d) The OH professional should advocate for keeping the employee in their current role regardless of their medical condition
e) The OH professional should advise on legal considerations regarding the dismissal of the employee

QUESTION 15

An employee has filed a grievance against her manager. Subsequently, she describes feeling ignored by her manager, which she feels is exacerbating her stress.

What one type of discrimination is she describing?

a) Direct discrimination
b) Harassment
c) Indirect discrimination
d) Unlawful dismissal
e) Victimisation

QUESTION 16

You are teaching a group of occupational health students about the legal responsibilities of employers under the Health and Safety at Work etc. Act 1974. You want to ensure that the students understand the key concepts related to the duties of employers in managing workplace risks.

Under the Health and Safety at Work etc. Act, what is the key concept that best outlines the duties of employers in managing workplace risks?

a) So far as is reasonably practicable (SFARP)
b) As low as reasonably practicable (ALARP)
c) Risk assessment
d) Hazard identification
e) Zero risk tolerance

QUESTION 17

Maria is a worker at a battery manufacturing plant where she is regularly exposed to lead. To ensure her safety and monitor her exposure levels, her employer conducts routine biological monitoring.

For biological monitoring of inorganic lead exposure, sampling is most typically performed using which one of the following?

a) Blood
b) Urine
c) Exhaled breath
d) Sweat
e) Hair

QUESTION 18

An employee has recently been diagnosed with Parkinson's disease. The condition currently has minimal effect on their work and daily life.

In which one of the following ways should this diagnosis be treated under the Equality Act 2010?

a) The employee should not be considered as having a disability until the Parkinson's disease starts to substantially affect their work and daily life
b) The employee should be treated as having a disability only if the Parkinson's disease causes noticeable difficulties in their work or daily life
c) The employee should be considered as having a disability now due to the progressive nature of Parkinson's disease, even if it currently has minimal impact

d) The employee should be provided with accommodations only if the Parkinson's disease is expected to affect their work in the near future
e) The employee's condition should be considered a disability only if they require specific workplace adjustments due to their Parkinson's disease

QUESTION 19

A 40-year-old oncology nurse is involved in the care of patients receiving radiation therapy. During a training session, the nurse asks which type of cells in the human body are most vulnerable to the effects of radiation. The nurse is particularly concerned about how radiation might affect different tissues in the body.

Which of the following cell types is most radiosensitive and therefore most at risk for radiation damage?

a) Neurons
b) Muscle cells
c) Lymphocytes
d) Bone cells
e) Liver cells

QUESTION 20

You are assisting an employer as an independent consultant to acquire occupational health services. You are asked whether Safe, Effective, Quality Occupational Health Service (SEQOHS) accreditation is needed for the service.

What is the most appropriate answer?

a) SEQOHS accreditation is a UK voluntary requirement
b) SEQOHS accreditation is a UK legal requirement
c) SEQOHS accreditation is a European voluntary requirement
d) SEQOHS accreditation is a European legal requirement
e) SEQOHS accreditation is a marker of international best practice

QUESTION 21

You are reviewing the skin surveillance system for a large hairdressing chain. All employees have completed a baseline high-level health surveillance questionnaire and visual inspection, but follow-up surveillance has not been conducted for two years.

When should the follow-up surveillance have been conducted for these employees?

a) At 6 weeks, 12 weeks, and then annually
b) At 3 months and then annually
c) Only when symptoms are reported
d) Annually
e) Every 6 months after the baseline assessment

QUESTION 22

You see a 29-year-old warehouse operator with non-specific upper limb pain who has been absent from work for 4 weeks.

What is the best intervention to help him to return to work?

a) Cognitive behavioural therapy aimed at improving coping mechanisms
b) Physiotherapy, with graded activity, aimed at increasing strength and endurance
c) Multidisciplinary rehabilitation including both physical and psychosocial approaches
d) Over-the-counter pain relief to facilitate increased function and improve comfort
e) TENS machine

QUESTION 23

You are an occupational health specialist conducting a workplace visit at a farm where employees regularly handle various farm animals. During your visit, you discuss zoonotic diseases and workplace safety with the farm manager.

Which one of the following legislations specifically applies to the risk assessment of zoonoses and their control measures in the workplace?

a) COSHH (Control of Substances Hazardous to Health Regulations) 2002
b) HASAWA (Health and Safety at Work etc. Act) 1974
c) Management of Health and Safety at Work Regulations 1999
d) Public Health (Control of Disease) Act 1984
e) Health Protection (Notification) Regulations 2010

QUESTION 24

During a training session for healthcare professionals you are discussing the importance of safeguarding patient information. A colleague asks about the purpose of the Caldicott Principles and their relevance to sharing information within health and social care settings.

Which of the following best describes the primary purpose of the Caldicott Principles?

a) To promote unrestricted sharing of patient records to ensure timely care
b) To inform good information sharing while protecting the confidentiality of patient records
c) To standardise the legal framework for health information sharing
d) To prioritise confidentiality over information sharing in all circumstances
e) To ensure patient consent is obtained for all data sharing

QUESTION 25

You are assessing a 50-year-old gardener who shows you photos of a linear rash on sun-exposed areas of their skin. The rash has led to significant post-inflammatory pigmentation where the marks previously were. The management team are seeking advice on managing their condition.

What is the most likely diagnosis?

a) Allergic contact dermatitis
b) Burns
c) Non-accidental injury
d) Dermatitis artefacta
e) Phytophotodermatitis

QUESTION 26

A 36-year-old employee has been managing long-term depression with counselling, which allows her to perform normal day-to-day activities effectively. Her employer seeks advice on whether the Equality Act 2010 is likely to apply in this case.

Under the Equality Act 2010, how should the impact of the employee's depression best be assessed to determine if it qualifies as a disability?

a) The Equality Act only applies if the employee is unable to perform day-to-day activities, even with treatment
b) The Equality Act does not apply because the employee can perform day-to-day activities due to treatment
c) The Equality Act applies only if the condition has lasted, or is expected to last, at least 12 months
d) The effect of treatment is disregarded when assessing whether the condition has a substantial adverse effect on day-to-day activities
e) The Equality Act applies only to physical impairments, not mental health impairments

QUESTION 27

You are involved in setting up a health surveillance programme for vibration exposure in a construction company about to commence operations. The company has a tight budget and wants to know who the most cost-effective person might be to administer tier 2 questionnaires.

What is the most appropriate option?

a) A responsible person
b) An appointed doctor
c) An Occupational Health nurse
d) Any employee
e) The most senior manager

QUESTION 28

You are an occupational health physician remotely assessing a 50-year-old receptionist who recently underwent an uncomplicated total abdominal hysterectomy. She is eager to return to work and her employer seeks advice on when it might be appropriate to do so.

Based on current guidelines, when are most women able to return to work after an uncomplicated total abdominal hysterectomy?

a) Most women are able to return to work by 4 weeks after an uncomplicated abdominal hysterectomy, depending on their recovery
b) Most women are able to return to work by 6–8 weeks after an uncomplicated abdominal hysterectomy, depending on their recovery
c) Most women are able to return to work by 10 weeks after an uncomplicated abdominal hysterectomy, depending on their recovery
d) Most women are able to return to work by 12 weeks after an uncomplicated abdominal hysterectomy, depending on their recovery
e) Most women are able to return to work by 16 weeks after an uncomplicated abdominal hysterectomy, depending on their recovery

QUESTION 29

You are undertaking a workplace visit to a bottling plant. You undertake a one-off noise reading as you have found it to be very noisy. The reading is 98 dB(A). Workers are not wearing any PPE and there are no signs to indicate that this is a restricted area.

What is the most appropriate next step?

a) Advise health surveillance for all workers
b) Advise a formal noise survey
c) Advise that all work needs to stop immediately
d) Advise that PPE is needed
e) Inform the HSE of a breach of regulations

QUESTION 30

You see a pregnant employee with a complicated pregnancy. She enquires about her rights regarding time off for antenatal (pregnancy-related) appointments.

Which one of the following statements about time off for antenatal appointments is correct?

a) Pregnant employees are not entitled to any paid leave for antenatal appointments
b) Pregnant employees are entitled to paid time off for antenatal appointments

c) Pregnant employees are entitled to paid leave for antenatal appointments but must make up the time lost
d) Pregnant employees are entitled to paid leave for up to three antenatal appointments, with any additional appointments requiring unpaid leave
e) Pregnant employees must take annual leave for antenatal appointments, as there is no entitlement to paid leave for these appointments

QUESTION 31

You are conducting a training session for Diploma students on workplace safety. During the session, you explain the importance of conducting risk assessments to identify potential hazards. One of the employees asks how risk is calculated in the context of a risk assessment and risk matrices.

Which of the following best describes how risk is calculated?

a) Risk = Severity × Frequency
b) Risk = Likelihood + Severity
c) Risk = Likelihood × Severity
d) Risk = Frequency × Impact
e) Risk = Likelihood × Impact + Severity

QUESTION 32

You are an occupational health doctor conducting a health assessment for Mr Patel, a 40-year-old worker in the construction industry. He has been exposed to respirable crystalline silica (RCS) for 15 years. You review his respiratory questionnaire and lung function tests, which are unremarkable.

What further investigation does Mr Patel most require as part of health surveillance for silica exposure?

a) Chest X-ray
b) Covid test
c) CT scan
d) Mantoux test
e) All of the above

Questions for Mock exam 2

QUESTION 33

You see a new receptionist in the radiology department who is worried about the risk of cancer from radiation exposure.

Which of the following is the most appropriate for the effect she is describing?

a) Deterministic effect
b) Hereditary effect
c) Late-onset effect
d) Random effect
e) Stochastic effect

QUESTION 34

You are conducting a workplace visit to a bakery that is monitoring the flour concentration as part of their risk monitoring process. The exposure is measured over two key time periods: long-term and short-term.

What are the two time periods used to measure workplace exposure limits (WELs) in the UK?

a) 8 hours (long-term) and 30 minutes (short-term)
b) 6 hours (long-term) and 15 minutes (short-term)
c) 8 hours (long-term) and 15 minutes (short-term)
d) 12 hours (long-term) and 30 minutes (short-term)
e) 6 hours (long-term) and 30 minutes (short-term)

QUESTION 35

You are evaluating a study that examines the mortality rates among workers exposed to a specific occupational hazard. In this study, the researchers use the general population as a comparison group to mortality. The results show that the workers have a lower observed mortality risk compared to the general population.

What type of bias may be having the most influence on the study's findings?

a) Selection bias
b) Information bias

c) Confounding bias
d) Healthy worker effect
e) Recall bias

QUESTION 36

You see Mx Jessop, a 45-year-old employee with substance misuse concerns. The employee disagrees with your opinion that they are fit to return to work with adjustments. Subsequently, the employer calls you after receiving a message from your administrator that they will not receive a report as the employee has withdrawn consent. The manager explains that she has paid for the report and is unable to further manage the employee's erratic absences without it.

What is the most appropriate course of action for you to take in this situation?

a) Advise the employer to contact the employee directly for further information
b) Explain that the employer needs to manage the case with the information that they already have
c) Explain the reason why the employee withdrew consent
d) Explain to the employer that no further information can be disclosed without the employee's consent
e) Send a summary report to the employer without the employee's consent, focusing only on your opinion

QUESTION 37

A 65-year-old construction worker presents with concerns about progressive contracture of his fingers. On examination, you observe thickening and shortening of the palmar fascia with noticeable contracture in his fingers.

Which of the following statements about Dupuytren's disease (DD) is most accurate?

a) Dupuytren's disease is more common in women
b) Dupuytren's disease is associated with conditions such as diabetes
c) Dupuytren's disease is associated with sun exposure
d) Dupuytren's disease has no genetic component
e) Dupuytren's disease is equally prevalent across different age groups

QUESTION 38

You are an occupational health advisor at a medium-sized manufacturing company. An employee has been on sick leave due to illness, and approaches you to discuss the company's policy on providing documentation for their absence. They are unsure about the requirements after being off work for more than a week.

Which one of the following would be the most appropriate for you to inform the employee regarding the requirement for a 'fit note' (sick note)?

a) The employee must provide a 'fit note' only if they have been absent for more than 10 working days
b) A 'fit note' is required if the employee has been ill and off work for more than 7 consecutive days
c) The employee is only required to provide a 'fit note' if they are absent for more than 14 consecutive days
d) A 'fit note' must be submitted for any period of illness, regardless of the duration of the absence
e) The employee does not need to provide any documentation unless specifically requested by their employer

QUESTION 39

At a bustling construction site a team is focused on concrete cutting and drilling operations on the ground floor.

The construction manager, concerned about the potential health hazards posed by airborne dust generated during these activities, has implemented a wet spray dust suppression system.

Which term best describes this type of control?

a) Elimination
b) Substitution
c) Engineering
d) Administrative
e) PPE

QUESTION 40

You are the occupational health advisor for a company that employs several night shift workers. The management team is reviewing its policies regarding health assessments for night workers. One of the managers asks you if employees are required to undergo health assessments before starting night work.

Which of the following is the most accurate response regarding the requirement for night workers to undergo health assessments?

a) Night workers are legally required to undergo a health assessment before starting night work
b) Night workers are legally required to attend health assessments in England only
c) Night workers must be offered a health assessment before starting night work, but they are not obligated to accept it
d) Night workers must attend an initial health assessment, but can decline follow-up assessments
e) Night workers are legally required to undergo regular health assessments

QUESTION 41

During a workplace visit to a film studio, you notice that the general lighting appears poor.

Which one of the following potential costs to the business is most likely to result from inadequate lighting?

a) Reduced productivity
b) Increased absenteeism
c) Reduced staff performance
d) Time off work because of accidents and injuries
e) All of the above

QUESTION 42

You see an individual with long Covid who has been absent from work for 6 months. The employer would like advice on the likelihood of return to work.

Based on general guidance, what is estimated likelihood of return to work?

a) 10%
b) 20%
c) 30%
d) 40%
e) 50%

QUESTION 43

You are teaching an occupational health trainee about safety-critical tasks.

Which of the following best defines a safety-critical task?

a) A task that requires employees to work with hazardous materials and follow strict safety protocols
b) A task that is very hazardous that could lead to significant personal injury or property damage
c) A task where personal impairment or error can jeopardise the safety of others or lead to a critical incident
d) A task where the use of personal protective equipment is enforced
e) A task that requires high levels of concentration and skill

QUESTION 44

You are planning a health promotion session for construction workers. You have been asked to focus on the main occupational health risks of construction work.

According to the HSE, what is the main risk to health that construction workers encounter?

a) Asbestos
b) Pitch
c) Silica
d) Ultraviolet (UV) light
e) Vibration

Questions and Answers for the Diploma in Occupational Medicine

QUESTION 45

You are an occupational health professional assessing the potential health effects of whole body vibration (WBV) on a group of heavy machinery operators.

Which of the following health effects is most commonly associated with WBV exposure?

a) Increased risk of cardiovascular disease
b) Increased risk of cervical spine disorders
c) Increased risk of gastrointestinal disorders
d) Increased risk of lumbar spine disease
e) All of the above

QUESTION 46

During a workplace visit to a construction site with 100 employees, you request to see the accident book, but the employer does not have one.

What is the most appropriate action regarding the employer's legal obligations?

a) Inform the employer that it would be beneficial to have an accident book to inform their future risk assessments
b) Advise the employer that they must purchase or create an accident book in case the HSE does an inspection
c) Advise the employer that they must purchase or create an accident book as required by law and keep it to record all workplace incidents
d) Notify the employer that they are only required to keep records if requested by their insurance company
e) Advise the employer that there is no need for an accident book

QUESTION 47

You are conducting a workplace visit at a construction site where cement is being used extensively. During the visit, you notice a worker kneeling in wet cement without proper protective gear. The worker appears unaware of the potential dangers associated with wet cement exposure.

Which option best describes the occupational health risks of exposure to wet cement?

a) Skin burns
b) Allergic dermatitis
c) Irritant dermatitis
d) Ocular chemical burns
e) All of the above

QUESTION 48

During a routine health assessment, you discover that an employee, who operates heavy machinery, has developed a severe health condition that could impair their ability to work safely. The employee insists that you do not disclose this information to their employer due to fear of losing their job. You are aware that disclosing this information could prevent potential harm to other employees and the public.

What are the most important aspects to consider when deciding whether to disclose this information in the public interest?

a) The patient's consent and their fear of losing their job
b) The severity and nature of the health condition and the risk it poses to others
c) The legal implications of breaching patient confidentiality
d) The employee's length of service and work performance history
e) The possibility of transferring the employee to a less risky role without disclosing the condition

QUESTION 49

A 34-year-old woman, who is applying for a promotion, discloses to her manager that she had severe depression when she was 18. The condition had a substantial and long-term adverse effect on her ability to carry out normal day-to-day activities at the time, but she has fully recovered and has not experienced any recurrence. The employer expresses concern about her past mental illness and is hesitant to promote her based on this information.

Under the Equality Act 2010, which one of the following statements is true regarding her protection against discrimination in this situation?

a) She is no longer protected under the Act because her condition is no longer present
b) She is protected under the Act as a person with a past disability
c) She is protected under the Act only if she has had a recurrence of her condition
d) She is protected under the Act only if she discloses her condition during the hiring process
e) She is protected under the Act only if her condition was symptomatic within the last 5 years

QUESTION 50

A 30-year-old worker with epilepsy accepts a job offer to operate heavy machinery in a manufacturing plant. The job involves working around unguarded moving parts and heights, where sudden loss of consciousness could result in serious injury. The worker does not disclose their medical condition to the employer during the pre-employment process. After a few weeks on the job, the worker has a seizure and is injured. An investigation into the incident raises concerns about whether the employee fulfilled their legal obligations under health and safety law.

Under the Health and Safety at Work etc. Act 1974 (HASAWA), which of the following statements best describes the employee's duties related to health and safety?

a) The employee has no obligation to disclose any medical conditions to the employer
b) The employee must disclose any relevant medical condition only if directly asked by the employer during the interview
c) The employee has a duty to take reasonable care of their own health and safety, which includes disclosing relevant medical conditions that could pose a hazard
d) The employee is only required to disclose relevant medical conditions that have already caused accidents in the workplace
e) The employee's duty to disclose medical conditions is voluntary and not legally required under the HASAWA

QUESTION 51

You review the blood lead levels for a 25-year-old woman. They are 25 μg/dl.

Reference values:

Action level – a blood lead concentration of:

- 25 μg/dl in a woman of reproductive capacity
- 40 μg/dl in a young person
- 50 μg/dl in any other employee

Suspension level – a blood lead concentration of:

- 30 μg/dl in a woman of reproductive capacity
- 50 μg/dl in a young person
- 60 μg/dl in any other employee

What should you advise the employer to be the most appropriate next step?

a) Carry out an urgent investigation to find out why this has happened
b) Report the result to the HSE
c) Stop work processes immediately
d) Suspend the employee
e) Stop the employee from doing work processes that expose her to lead

QUESTION 52

You encounter a 35-year-old baker presenting with symptoms suggestive of occupational asthma. Spirometry reveals an obstructive pattern.

Which is the most appropriate investigation to establish a diagnosis?

a) Chest X-ray
b) Bronchial provocation challenge
c) Serial peak flows
d) Further spirometry
e) Workplace challenge

QUESTION 53

You see a 40-year-old psychiatry registrar who is currently 30 weeks pregnant. She works in a sedentary role with minimal manual handling and works up to 50 hours a week. As part of her revised pregnancy risk assessment, her employer wishes to reduce her working hours. The employee wishes to continue working as usual until she starts her maternity leave.

What is the most appropriate advice to give her employer?

a) As the Equality Act applies, she is entitled to work as she pleases
b) Her hours should be limited to 40 per week in late pregnancy if possible
c) She can continue to work long hours if she wishes, with an understanding of the risks
d) She should be medically restricted from working long hours
e) She should be redeployed to a role with shorter hours for the rest of her pregnancy

QUESTION 54

You are working with the safety team who have performed a risk assessment requiring the use of half mask respirators in environments with silica dust.

What is the most appropriate next step the employer should take to ensure optimal control is provided when implementing this change?

a) Conduct health surveillance
b) Ensure appropriate storage
c) Fit test
d) Perform dust monitoring
e) Provide information on how to use the mask

QUESTION 55

You are visiting a farm on a workplace visit. When talking to a sheep farmer, you notice a lesion on her finger. She tells you that this started as a reddish-blue lump which enlarged to a flat-topped, blood-tinged pustule about 2–3 cm across. She says it is painless.

What is the most likely diagnosis?

a) Anthrax
b) Cowpox
c) Herpetic whitlow
d) Milker's nodule
e) Orf

QUESTION 56

Reported cases of toxoplasmosis in the UK are fairly rare. However, it is estimated that up to a third of the population are infected with *Toxoplasma gondii* at some time in their lives.

From the list below, which animal is most likely to spread this infection?

a) Cows
b) Cats
c) Dogs
d) Parrots
e) Pigeons

QUESTION 57

During a workplace visit in an office, you notice that it is quite cold even on a summer's day, and many employees are still wearing their coats.

Under the Workplace (Health, Safety and Welfare) Regulations 1992 and considering the diversity in personal comfort levels, what is the minimum temperature guideline for maintaining a comfortable office environment?

a) A minimum of 13°C for sedentary work
b) A minimum of 16°C for sedentary work
c) It depends on whether it is summer or winter
d) There is no minimum temperature specification
e) This should be based on the group of employees' preference

QUESTION 58

You are asked to help set up a biological monitoring system at a yacht building company working with styrene. A biological monitoring guidance value (BMGV) is set at 1 micromol (1 µmol) urinary diamine per mol creatinine. You are asked what is likely to happen if employees have values above this level.

What is the most appropriate answer?

a) The business will have breached legislation
b) The employees are likely to have ill-health effects of exposure to styrene
c) The business is not following best practice
d) Work practices and controls need to be investigated
e) The employees have not been using the controls in place

QUESTION 59

You are undertaking a workplace visit at a gardening company with students. One of your students asks you what the limit value for hand arm vibration is.

What is the most appropriate answer?

a) 0.5 m/s^2 A(8)
b) 1.15 m/s^2 A(8)
c) 2.5 m/s^2 A(8)
d) 4.5 m/s^2 (A)8
e) 5.0 m/s^2 A(8)

QUESTION 60

A manager notices that several employees have been coming to work despite being ill and performing below their usual standards. This decline in performance has affected overall productivity in the team.

What is the most appropriate term to describe this phenomenon?

a) Absenteeism
b) Presenteeism
c) Job burnout
d) Work–life imbalance
e) Overtime

QUESTION 61

A worker complains of eye discomfort and distraction while working on a computer screen for long periods in a brightly lit office. The lighting in the room causes a part of the visual field to be much brighter than the rest. Although the worker's vision is not directly impaired, they report feeling irritated and visually fatigued.

Which term best describes the glare this worker is experiencing?

a) Disability glare
b) Visual field glare
c) Discomfort glare
d) Fatigue-induced glare
e) Reflex glare

QUESTION 62

You see a student midwife who has just started her clinical rotation. She was in the birthing suite when she noticed a burning sensation and red swellings on her hands. The rash resolved itself within 24 hours of onset.

You suspect that this was related to wearing latex gloves.

What is the most likely type of reaction in this condition?

a) Type 1 hypersensitivity
b) Type 2 hypersensitivity
c) Type 3 hypersensitivity
d) Type 4 hypersensitivity
e) Type 5 hypersensitivity

QUESTION 63

You receive a call from an occupational technician who is on site undertaking pure tone audiometry as part of routine health surveillance assessment for noise exposure. He describes an audiogram for a 45-year-old factory worker attending for his 3-year review; the summation of the hearing levels obtained at 1, 2, 3, 4 and 6 kHz indicates a new Category 3 result in both ears.

What action would it be most appropriate to take, based on this result?

a) Arrange a repeat audiometry in 6 months
b) Conduct a workplace noise assessment
c) Provide ear protection training
d) Further review by an OHP
e) Refer the employee to an ENT specialist

QUESTION 64

Oskar applies for a job as a scaffolder. On the application form, he is asked whether there is any reason why he cannot climb ladders or work at a height, both tasks intrinsic to the job. Oskar discloses that he has epilepsy, which he manages with medication. The employer is concerned about the safety implications of Oskar working at heights and decides to conduct a risk assessment to determine if the work is hazardous for him.

As an occupational health physician advising the employer, what is the best course of action to ensure compliance with the Equality Act 2010 while addressing the safety concerns?

a) Advise that the employer cannot ask questions about an employee's health prior to a job offer, as rejection may be deemed discriminatory
b) Advise that, as Oskar would be deemed disabled under the Equality Act, he must be given reasonable adjustments to do the role
c) Conduct a thorough risk assessment to determine if there are reasonable adjustments that could enable Oskar to safely perform the job
d) Instruct the employer to hire Oskar but exclude him from tasks involving heights to ensure his safety
e) Recommend that the employer reject Oskar's application due to the inherent safety risks, without conducting a risk assessment

QUESTION 65

You conduct a walkthrough survey at a mechanics shop and ask to see the risk assessment, but the employer does not have one documented.

How many employees does an employer need to have before there is a legal requirement to document a risk assessment?

a) 2
b) 3
c) 5
d) 10
e) 15

QUESTION 66

A company is developing a strategy to manage and reduce employee absenteeism.

Which of the following statements best reflects the importance of past sickness absence?

a) Past sickness absence is not a reliable predictor of future absence risk
b) Past sickness absence is a key indicator of future absence risk, with a higher number of past absences suggesting an increased risk of future absences
c) Past sickness absence only affects future absence risk if it occurs within the same calendar year
d) Past sickness absence has a minimal impact on predicting future absence risk compared to other factors
e) Employees with past sickness absences are less likely to experience future absences if they have had a period of consistent attendance

QUESTION 67

A warehouse packer who suffers from Raynaud's disease complains that the warehouse is too cold.

What is the minimum temperature requirement for this workplace?

a) 9°C
b) 13°C
c) 15°C
d) 17°C
e) 19°C

QUESTION 68

You are an occupational health advisor for a manufacturing company where employees are frequently exposed to metal fumes from welding. The company is considering offering pneumococcal vaccinations to all employees to reduce the risk of pneumococcal diseases. Some employees have expressed concerns about the vaccine and are unsure if they want to receive it.

What is the most appropriate advice to provide the company regarding the pneumococcal vaccination policy for employees exposed to metal fumes?

a) The company should make the pneumococcal vaccine mandatory for all employees exposed to metal fumes, to ensure maximum protection
b) Employees who refuse the pneumococcal vaccine should be redeployed away from tasks involving metal fume exposure, to protect their health and safety
c) Employees should be strongly encouraged to take the pneumococcal vaccine to minimise workplace health risks, and refusal should be documented in their personnel files
d) Only employees who express interest should be given detailed information about the pneumococcal vaccine, to avoid unnecessary concerns among others
e) The pneumococcal vaccine should be presented as optional for employees, with assurance that they will not face any negative consequences if they choose not to receive it

QUESTION 69

You see a student nurse in your screening clinic who is due to start work on the paediatric ward. As part of routine screening, you note that her interferon gamma release assay (IGRA) test is negative but she has not been vaccinated against tuberculosis (TB).

Which one of the following is the most appropriate next step prior to BCG vaccination?

a) HIV test
b) Mantoux test
c) Chest X-ray

d) CT
e) HR-CT

QUESTION 70

A healthcare worker sustains a needlestick injury while treating a patient known to be positive for hepatitis B.

What is the estimated risk of hepatitis B transmission from the patient to the healthcare worker?

a) Up to 1%
b) Up to 30%
c) 5–10%
d) 1–3%
e) 0.3%

QUESTION 71

You are helping a student with a research problem. They have some queries about confidence intervals.

If a study quotes a 95% confidence interval, which one of the following statements is true?

a) There is a 95% chance of the true value lying outside these limits
b) There is a 5% chance of the true value lying outside these limits
c) There is a 2.5% chance of the true value lying outside these limits
d) There is a minus 5% chance of the true value lying outside these limits
e) None of the above

QUESTION 72

You are an occupational health physician for a corporate office. You see Ms Floyd, a data analyst who works long hours at a computer. She complains of frequent eye strain, headaches and neck discomfort. Ms Floyd mentions that due to her workload, she often skips breaks and continues working at her desk for extended periods without interruption.

Based on Ms Floyd's symptoms and the regulations concerning display screen equipment (DSE) users, what is the most appropriate advice you should provide regarding breaks?

a) Breaks should be taken when directed by break-monitoring software
b) Breaks should be determined by the employer based on the business requirements and deadlines
c) Short breaks taken frequently are more beneficial than longer breaks less often
d) The legal requirement is 15 to 20 minutes every hour
e) The legal requirement is a 20-minute break every 4 hours as a minimum

QUESTION 73

You are an occupational health physician who has been asked to provide evidence for an employment tribunal regarding a case where a worker alleges unfair dismissal due to a disability. Your role involves providing expert opinions on the worker's health and its impact on their employment.

What is the primary function of the employment tribunal in this context?

a) To adjudicate criminal cases related to workplace safety violations
b) To offer mediation services to resolve disputes between employees and employers
c) To make legally binding decisions on disputes related to employment rights
d) To provide counselling and support services to employees experiencing workplace stress
e) To conduct workplace inspections and ensure compliance with health and safety regulations

QUESTION 74

A 50-year-old radiation safety officer is conducting a training session for new staff at a hospital that uses various types of radiological equipment. The officer needs to explain the different penetrating potentials of radiation types, to ensure that appropriate safety measures and shielding are in place. The staff ask for clarification on which type of radiation requires the most substantial shielding due to its high penetrating power.

Which of the following types of radiation has the greatest penetrating ability and therefore requires the most substantial shielding?

a) Alpha particles
b) Beta particles
c) Gamma rays
d) X-rays
e) Positrons

QUESTION 75

You see a 50-year-old farmer with a 3-month history of cough and shortness of breath that he feels is worse at work. His symptoms improved during a recent 3-week holiday. He also reports malaise and weight loss. He does not smoke and has an otherwise unremarkable medical history.

What is the most likely diagnosis?

a) Chronic obstructive pulmonary disease (COPD)
b) Hypersensitivity pneumonitis (HP)
c) Lung cancer
d) Obliterative bronchiolitis
e) Occupational asthma

QUESTION 76

You are an occupational health professional starting a new role at a large healthcare organisation. As part of your induction, you are informed about the safeguarding training requirements necessary for your role. The organisation highlights the importance of ensuring that all staff working in occupational health are appropriately trained to identify and act on safeguarding concerns involving children and vulnerable individuals.

What is the minimum level of safeguarding training required for occupational health professionals?

a) Level 1 safeguarding training
b) Level 2 safeguarding training
c) Level 3 safeguarding training
d) Level 4 safeguarding training
e) Safeguarding training is not required for occupational health professionals

QUESTION 77

You have been asked to review a spirometry test performed by a student technician for asbestos health surveillance, and the results are shown in the graph below.

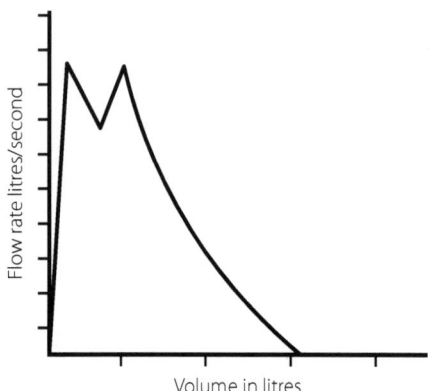

What is the most likely cause of the spirometry pattern observed in this graph?

a) Cough during the test
b) Extra breath taken during the test
c) Obstructive lung disease
d) Restrictive lung disease
e) Suboptimal technique

QUESTION 78

You see a 42-year-old construction worker who has worked with pneumatic drills for 1 year. He is complaining of numbness and tingling in the little and ring finger of his dominant hand, which he feels is associated with using the drill. He does notice that it also occurs when he is lifting weights at the gym. He is a smoker of 10 cigarettes a day since he was 20 years old.

From the information above, what is the most likely diagnosis?

a) Carpal tunnel syndrome
b) Cubital tunnel syndrome
c) Hand arm vibration syndrome
d) Raynaud's disease
e) Thoracic outlet syndrome

QUESTION 79

You are an NHS occupational health physician. You are evaluating a hospital porter and need more information to guide your decision-making regarding his fitness for work. You notice that he is currently under the care of several specialists at the hospital where you work.

What is the best way to obtain the information that you need?

a) Access the hospital porter's medical records directly to obtain the necessary information
b) Request information from the specialists directly without informing the patient
c) Contact the specialists and request the necessary information, copying the hospital porter on the communication
d) Obtain the hospital porter's consent to request information from his specialists
e) Make a fitness-for-work decision based on the information already provided without seeking further details

QUESTION 80

You are writing hospital guidance for the management of healthcare workers who accidentally sustain needlestick injuries.

What is the most appropriate immediate action following the injury?

a) Scrub the wound thoroughly with soap and water to ensure all contaminants are removed
b) Suck the wound to remove any potential blood-borne pathogens
c) Gently encourage the wound to bleed and wash it with soap and water
d) Keep the needle for laboratory testing to check for blood-borne viruses
e) Re-sheath the needle and send it to the lab for testing

ANSWERS to Mock exam 2

QUESTION 1

A study is investigating the link between substance Y and lung cancer. Researchers find that individuals who worked in industries linked to substance Y exposure had a higher incidence of lung cancer. They want to use the Bradford Hill criteria to demonstrate an association.

Which of the following best defines the Bradford Hill criterion of temporality in this context?

The answer is: b) A demonstration that the cause precedes the effect

The Bradford Hill criteria used to determine causation:
- *Strength of association*: examines the magnitude of the relationship between exposure and disease. A stronger association (e.g. a high relative risk or odds ratio) lends more weight to the causal inference. If the exposure is strongly linked to the disease, it supports the likelihood of a causal relationship.
- *Temporality*: refers to whether the exposure precedes the onset of the disease. For a causal relationship, the exposure must occur before the disease develops. This is a fundamental criterion because if the disease occurs before the exposure, causation cannot be established.
- *Dose–response relationship*: assesses whether increasing levels of exposure result in a corresponding increase in the risk of the disease. A clear dose–response relationship supports causation, as it suggests that higher exposures lead to higher risks of disease, demonstrating a biological gradient.
- *Analogy*: involves comparing the exposure–disease relationship to similar known relationships in other contexts. If similar exposures have been shown to cause the same or similar diseases elsewhere, it supports the likelihood that the exposure in question might also be causative.

- *Consistency*: refers to whether the association between exposure and disease is observed across different studies, populations and settings. A consistent finding across various studies and conditions strengthens the evidence for a causal relationship.
- *Coherence*: examines whether the association makes sense within the broader context of existing knowledge about the disease and exposure. It checks if the findings are consistent with the known biology and other evidence related to the disease.
- *Specificity*: looks at whether the exposure is associated with a specific disease and not with other unrelated diseases. A high degree of specificity suggests that the exposure–disease relationship is causal, though this criterion is less commonly met in complex exposures.
- *Experiment*: involves evidence from experiments or interventions. If altering the exposure (e.g. through control measures or treatment) leads to changes in the incidence or prevalence of the disease, it supports the causal relationship. Experimental evidence can strengthen the case for causation.

Each of these criteria provides a different angle of evidence for evaluating causality, and collectively they help in assessing whether a particular exposure causes a disease.

QUESTION 2

You are conducting a workplace health and safety review for a large retailer. The employer is concerned about the risk of Covid-19 among employees and wants to identify individuals who may be more susceptible to severe outcomes if they contract the virus. You are asked to provide guidance on the factors that increase individual susceptibility to severe Covid-19 infection.

Which of the following is a factor that most increases individual susceptibility to severe Covid-19 infection?

The answer is: e) All of the above

Factors that increase individual susceptibility for severe Covid-19 infection include the following:
- Immunosuppressive treatment, such as for cancer treatment or autoimmune disorders
- Chronic conditions, e.g. lung and heart conditions, diabetes
- Older age (over 70 years)

- Pregnant women
- Obesity
- Black and Asian ethnicity.

Source: Sadhra, S., Bray, A.J. and Boorman, S. (eds) (2022) *Oxford Handbook of Occupational Health*, 3rd edition

QUESTION 3

You are consulted to provide guidance on which types of procedures pose a risk of transmitting blood-borne viruses (BBVs) from the healthcare worker (HCW) to the patient.

Which of the following best describes an exposure-prone procedure (EPP)?

The answer is: b) Procedures where the HCW's blood may contaminate the patient's open tissues if an injury occurs

Exposure-prone procedures (EPPs) are healthcare procedures where there is a risk that injury to the HCW may result in the exposure of the patient's open tissues to the blood of the worker (bleed-back). Procedures include those where the worker's gloved hands may be in contact with sharp instruments, needle tips, and sharp tissues (spicules of bone or teeth) inside a patient's open body cavity, wound, or confined anatomical space where the hands or fingertips may not be completely visible at all times.

The defining feature of EPPs is the potential for a HCW's blood to enter a patient's open tissues during a procedure, particularly if the HCW sustains an injury, making option b) the correct answer.

Sources:
- https://assets.publishing.service.gov.uk/media/5c40663ae5274a6e4f614dc1/general_surgery_exposure_prone_procedure_epp_categorisation.pdf
- Sadhra, S., Bray, A.J. and Boorman, S. (eds) (2022) *Oxford Handbook of Occupational Health*, 3rd edition

QUESTION 4

You are teaching occupational medicine trainees about identifying factors that could influence an individual's susceptibility to prolonged illness or sickness absence.

In the context of the flags system used for this purpose, which of the following is most appropriately considered a 'chequered flag'?

The answer is: e) Social factors such as caregiving responsibilities or other commitments outside of work

One way of segmenting obstacles to return to work may be to use a flag system.

These flags guide clinicians in identifying obstacles to recovery and ensuring appropriate support and interventions.
- *Red flags*: factors suggestive of serious medical pathology
- *Orange flags*: psychological disorders
- *Yellow flags*: individual factors impacting on perception, mood or beliefs; examples include catastrophising, and unhelpful beliefs about pain and work
- *Blue flags*: organisational issues and policies; examples include low job satisfaction and poor support at work
- *Black flags*: financial situation; an example would be threats to financial stability including the risk of litigation
- *Chequered flags*: represent social factors affecting an individual's ability to return to work and may need alternative employment options or flexible working arrangements.

Sources:
- Hobson, J. and Smedley, J. (eds) (2019) *Fitness for Work: the medical aspects*, 6th edition. Oxford University Press
- Sadhra, S., Bray, A.J. and Boorman, S. (eds) (2022) *Oxford Handbook of Occupational Health*, 3rd edition

QUESTION 5

You are working for a large office-based company with 10 000 employees. As a result of the Covid-19 pandemic, its employees are now all agile workers. The company wants to know how to fulfil its health and safety duties to employees working from home.

What is the most appropriate advice to give the employer?

The answer is: d) The employer should provide their employees with information to do a self-risk assessment of their home

By law, employers must conduct a 'suitable and sufficient' risk assessment of their employees' working environment. Undertaking a full risk assessment from home is unlikely to be realistic for a large company. If an employer is not able to carry out a full risk assessment, they should provide their employees with information on working safely at home. This could include asking them to carry out a self-assessment of their workspace and equipment. Employees must report all employment-related hazards to their employer and ensure that their homeworking environment stays suitable and appropriate in line with the workplace health and safety risk assessment.

The employer and employee should check insurance and other considerations to ensure that home working is a viable option, but the most appropriate next step to ensure that their health and safety duties are fulfilled is to undertake a risk assessment.

QUESTION 6

During an annual review of anonymised health surveillance audiometric results, it is observed that there has been a deterioration in hearing among a specific group of workers.

What is the most appropriate next step in response to these findings?

The answer is: b) Reassess the exposure factors to identify potential changes in exposure conditions that may have contributed to the deterioration

If there is deterioration in hearing, simply continuing with current measures without investigation may not address potential underlying issues.

Reassessing exposure factors is crucial to determine if changes in noise exposure conditions, such as machinery relocation or inadequate maintenance, could be contributing to the hearing deterioration.

While reassessing the workers' hearing is important, the immediate next step should focus on identifying and addressing changes in exposure conditions that could be causing the deterioration.

While increased use of hearing protection might be necessary, the priority should be to understand and address any changes in exposure conditions that might be causing the deterioration.

Training is important, but the immediate focus should be on identifying and correcting any changes in exposure conditions that may be leading to the deterioration of hearing.

Source: www.hse.gov.uk/pubns/priced/l108.pdf

QUESTION 7

You are an occupational health and safety officer conducting a routine inspection at a manufacturing plant. During your visit, an employee mentions that they want to sign a disclaimer to opt out of wearing the required personal protective equipment (PPE) because they find it uncomfortable and believe the risk in their specific role is minimal. The employee asks if this is permissible.

What is the most appropriate response to the employee's request to sign a disclaimer to not wear PPE?

The answer is: d) Inform the employee that signing a disclaimer is not possible, as employers are legally required to provide PPE and ensure its use when risks cannot be controlled in other ways

Under health and safety regulations, PPE is required when there are risks to health and safety that cannot be adequately controlled by other means. Employees cannot sign a disclaimer to opt out of wearing PPE, as it is the employer's duty to ensure all employees use the necessary protective equipment. The use of PPE is a legal requirement to minimise exposure to hazards, and exemptions are not allowed based on personal discomfort or perceived low risk. The employer must also ensure that PPE is suitable, properly maintained, and used correctly by all employees.

Source: www.hse.gov.uk/stonemasonry/faqs.htm#reduce-vibration

QUESTION 8

You see an employee who has recently been diagnosed with occupational asthma by a respiratory physician. You are aware that this is a RIDDOR reportable disease.

Which of the following is required to submit reports of injuries, diseases and dangerous occurrences under RIDDOR?

The answer is: c) The responsible person

Answers to Mock exam 2

Under the Reporting of Injuries, Diseases and Dangerous Occurrences Regulations 2013 (RIDDOR), it is the responsibility of the 'responsible person' in the workplace to submit reports of injuries, diseases and dangerous occurrences. This includes employers, the self-employed, and those in control of work premises. The employee who has been diagnosed with occupational asthma is not required to submit the report themselves. Similarly, while the occupational physician may diagnose the condition, they are not responsible for filing the report. The manager is also not responsible for submitting the report. The onus is on the responsible person to ensure compliance with RIDDOR reporting requirements.

Source: www.hse.gov.uk/riddor/who-should-report.htm

QUESTION 9

You are an occupational health professional asked to review a group of office workers who have reported a variety of symptoms, including dry or itchy skin, dry or itchy eyes, nose or throat, headaches, lethargy and a runny nose. On examination, all individuals show normal physical findings. Recent inspections of the air conditioning and ventilation systems in the office building were unremarkable.

What is the most likely diagnosis for these workers?

The answer is: c) Sick building syndrome

Sick building syndrome (SBS) describes a situation where occupants of a building experience acute health symptoms that are associated with time spent in the building but with no specific illness or cause identified. The symptoms, such as dry or itchy skin, dry or itchy eyes, nose or throat, headaches, lethargy and a runny nose, are consistent with SBS. The fact that all workers are experiencing these symptoms while in the same environment, and the symptoms improve when away from the building, supports SBS as the most likely diagnosis.

Humidifier fever is caused by exposure to contaminated humidifiers or air conditioning systems and is characterised by flu-like symptoms such as fever, chills, muscle aches and malaise. The symptoms are more severe than those reported by the workers and usually include a fever, which is not mentioned in the scenario. Additionally, inspections of the air conditioning and ventilation systems were unremarkable, making this diagnosis less likely.

The common cold can present with some of the symptoms mentioned, such as a runny nose, headaches and lethargy. However, a cold would typically not cause symptoms such as dry or itchy skin or eyes, and it would be less likely to affect a group of workers simultaneously in the same environment without a known infectious outbreak. Moreover, a common cold would usually present with more upper respiratory symptoms such as a sore throat and cough.

Occupational asthma is a form of asthma triggered by inhaling fumes, gases, dust or other potentially harmful substances in the workplace. It often presents with respiratory symptoms such as coughing, wheezing, chest tightness and shortness of breath. The symptoms described in this scenario do not include respiratory complaints typical of asthma, making this diagnosis less likely.

Legionnaires' disease is a severe form of pneumonia caused by *Legionella* bacteria, commonly found in contaminated water systems. Symptoms typically include high fever, cough, shortness of breath, muscle aches and headaches, which are more severe than the mild symptoms reported by the workers. Additionally, the scenario mentions that recent inspections of air conditioning and ventilation systems were unremarkable, further ruling out this diagnosis.

Source: www.hse.gov.uk/pubns/priced/hsg132.pdf

QUESTION 10

You are conducting a consultation with an employee, and at the end of the session, they request a copy of their medical records. They ask how long it will take for them to receive this information once they make a formal request.

How long does an organisation have to provide the requested information after a formal Subject Access Request (SAR) is made?

The answer is: c) 1 month

Employees have the legal right to access their personal data, including medical records. Under the UK General Data Protection Regulation (UK GDPR), organisations are required to respond to a formal Subject Access Request (SAR) within one calendar month. This timeframe includes weekends and holidays, starting from the day the request is received. Extensions of up to an additional two months may be granted for complex requests, but this must be communicated to the requester within the original one-month period.

Source: https://ico.org.uk/for-the-public/getting-copies-of-your-information-subject-access-request

QUESTION 11

You are working with a manufacturer on their preventive health strategy. You note that a third of their workforce are welders.

Which vaccination is most appropriate to offer this workforce?

The answer is: d) Pneumococcal

Pneumococcal vaccination should be considered for welders, as they are at increased risk of pneumococcal pneumonia due to inhaling welding fumes. This vaccination can help mitigate that specific risk. Vaccination may reduce the risk of invasive pneumococcal disease but should not replace the need for measures to prevent or reduce exposure.

While Covid-19 vaccination is important for general public health, this vaccination does not specifically address the occupational hazards associated with welding.

Hepatitis B vaccination is relevant for those at risk of blood-borne pathogens, which is not a primary concern for welders.

Influenza vaccination helps prevent flu but does not address the specific occupational hazards related to welding.

Varicella zoster vaccination is for preventing chickenpox and shingles, which are not associated with welding hazards.

Source: www.hse.gov.uk/pubns/eis44.pdf

QUESTION 12

You are an OHP working in a manufacturing plant where employees are exposed to various hazardous materials. Your employer has asked you to review the need for statutory medical surveillance to ensure compliance with health and safety regulations. You note that the plant uses materials that involve exposure to lead, asbestos and ionising radiation.

Which one professional is specifically appointed by the Health and Safety Executive (HSE) to conduct statutory medical surveillance under specific regulations?

The answer is: b) Appointed Doctor

An Appointed Doctor is a registered medical practitioner appointed by the HSE to conduct statutory medical surveillance under specific regulations.

These include:
- Ionising Radiations Regulations 2017
- Control of Lead at Work Regulations 2002
- Control of Asbestos Regulations 2012
- Control of Substances Hazardous to Health Regulations 2002
- Work in Compressed Air Regulations 1996.

These professionals are required to ensure compliance with legal standards and to monitor the health of workers who are exposed to certain occupational hazards.

Source: www.hse.gov.uk/doctors/about.htm

QUESTION 13

An employer is reviewing their health and safety protocols for employees who work with ionising radiation.

Under radiation protection regulations, how are employees designated as 'classified persons' when working with ionising radiation?

The answer is: c) Employees are designated as classified persons if they are likely to receive a personal radiation dose exceeding 6 mSv per year

In the context of radiation protection regulations, employees who are likely to receive a personal annual dose of ionising radiation exceeding 6 mSv or 3/10ths of any other exposure limits are designated as 'classified persons'. This designation is important for ensuring that specific safety and monitoring and health surveillance measures are implemented to protect employees from excessive radiation exposure.

Source: www.bir.org.uk/media/495365/advice_sheet_4_classification_of_nuclear_medicine_staff_v2.pdf

QUESTION 14

You are an occupational health (OH) professional asked to assess an employee who has been off sick for a prolonged period. The manager seeks your opinion on whether the employee should be dismissed due to their inability to work.

Answers to Mock exam 2

What is the most appropriate role of the OH professional in this situation?

The answer is: c) The OH professional should provide and interpret medical information, allowing the employer to make an informed decision about dismissal

The decision to dismiss an employee is a managerial responsibility, not a medical one.

The OH professional should remain neutral and provide objective medical information rather than advocating for specific employment outcomes.

Legal advice should come from legal professionals, while the OH professional focuses on medical input.

Source: Hobson, J. and Smedley, J. (eds) (2019) *Fitness for Work: the medical aspects*, 6th edition. Oxford University Press

QUESTION 15

An employee has filed a grievance against her manager. Subsequently, she describes feeling ignored by her manager, which she feels is exacerbating her stress.

What one type of discrimination is she describing?

The answer is: e) Victimisation

The employee's feeling of being ignored after filing a grievance against her manager may suggest victimisation.

Victimisation occurs when someone is treated unfairly because they have taken action under the Equality Act, such as filing a grievance or other proceedings related to discrimination. This aligns with the employee's experience of adverse treatment following her grievance.

The Equality Act 2010 aims to prevent discrimination in the workplace. It is illegal to discriminate against workers based on nine protected characteristics.

The law covers four different types of discrimination: direct, indirect, harassment and victimisation.
- *Direct*: where a person discriminates against another because of one of these protected characteristics
- *Indirect*: where a person puts conditions in place that put another at a disadvantage because of one of the protected characteristics

- *Harassment*: where a person engages in unwanted conduct, creates an intimidating, hostile or offensive environment, or violates someone else's dignity in relation to a protected characteristic
- *Victimisation*: where someone treats another badly because they are taking part in or are thought to be taking part in proceedings related to the Equality Act.

The term 'unlawful dismissal' typically refers to wrongful termination of employment, which may involve a breach of contract or dismissal for discriminatory reasons. While the employee's situation involves adverse treatment following a grievance, it does not directly imply dismissal from her job. Therefore 'unlawful dismissal' is not the type of discrimination described in this scenario.

Source: www.acas.org.uk/discrimination-and-the-law/victimisation

QUESTION 16

You are teaching a group of occupational health students about the legal responsibilities of employers under the Health and Safety at Work etc. Act 1974. You want to ensure that the students understand the key concepts related to the duties of employers in managing workplace risks.

Under the Health and Safety at Work etc. Act, what is the key concept that best outlines the duties of employers in managing workplace risks?

The answer is: a) So far as is reasonably practicable (SFARP)

SFARP is the correct concept under the Health and Safety at Work etc. Act. It means that employers must take all reasonably practicable steps to ensure health and safety at work, considering the balance between the level of risk and the measures required to control it.

While closely related to SFARP, ALARP is more commonly used in risk management frameworks outside of the Health and Safety at Work etc. Act. It also implies reducing risks to a level that is as low as reasonably practicable, but is not the exact term used in the Act.

Risk assessment is a process that employers must undertake to identify and control risks. However, it is not the specific concept that defines the duties of employers under the Act.

Identifying hazards is an essential part of the risk assessment process, but is not the overarching concept that defines employers' duties under the Act.

Zero risk tolerance: this concept suggests eliminating all risks, which is not practical or required under the Health and Safety at Work etc. Act. The Act focuses on balancing risks with practicable measures, rather than achieving zero risk.

Source: www.legislation.gov.uk/ukpga/1974/37/section/2

QUESTION 17

Maria is a worker at a battery manufacturing plant where she is regularly exposed to lead. To ensure her safety and monitor her exposure levels, her employer conducts routine biological monitoring.

For biological monitoring of inorganic lead exposure, sampling is most typically performed using which one of the following?

The answer is: a) Blood

For biological monitoring of lead exposure:
- *Inorganic lead*: blood lead concentration is measured. It reflects recent exposure and is influenced by factors such as air lead concentration, physical properties of lead compounds, working practices and personal hygiene. In cases of low current exposure, blood lead levels may also be affected by the mobilisation of lead from bone.
- *Organic lead*: total lead in urine is measured. This method reflects exposure to both organic and inorganic lead.

Source: www.hse.gov.uk/pubns/ms40.pdf

QUESTION 18

An employee has recently been diagnosed with Parkinson's disease. The condition currently has minimal effect on their work and daily life.

In which one of the following ways should this diagnosis be treated under the Equality Act 2010?

The answer is: c) The employee should be considered as having a disability now due to the progressive nature of Parkinson's disease, even if it currently has minimal impact

The Equality Act provides that where an individual has a progressive condition which is likely to have a substantial adverse effect on the individual's normal day-to-day activities at some future stage, then that condition is to be treated as having such a substantial adverse effect now, even if it has yet to do so.

Parkinson's disease, being a progressive condition, should be treated as if it currently has a substantial adverse effect. This approach ensures that the employee receives necessary accommodations and support in anticipation of future needs, adhering to the principles of equality and prevention.

Accommodations should be considered based on the potential future impact of the condition, not just immediate effects. Waiting until the condition affects work may lead to unnecessary difficulties for the employee.

The recognition of a disability should not be contingent upon immediate need for accommodations. The progressive nature of Parkinson's disease necessitates early recognition and proactive support.

Source: Hobson, J. and Smedley, J. (eds) (2019) *Fitness for Work: the medical aspects*, 6th edition. Oxford University Press

QUESTION 19

A 40-year-old oncology nurse is involved in the care of patients receiving radiation therapy. During a training session, the nurse asks which type of cells in the human body are most vulnerable to the effects of radiation. The nurse is particularly concerned about how radiation might affect different tissues in the body.

Which of the following cell types is most radiosensitive and therefore most at risk for radiation damage?

The answer is: c) Lymphocytes

Lymphocytes are the most radiosensitive cells due to their high mitotic rate and minimal differentiation. This makes them particularly vulnerable to radiation, which can cause significant DNA damage and impair their function. These cells are more resistant to radiation because they are highly specialised and rarely divide.

While bone cells can be affected by radiation, they are less sensitive compared to lymphocytes.

Although liver cells have some regenerative capacity, they are still less radiosensitive than lymphocytes.

QUESTION 20

You are assisting an employer as an independent consultant to acquire occupational health services. You are asked whether Safe, Effective, Quality Occupational Health Service (SEQOHS) accreditation is needed for the service.

What is the most appropriate answer?

The answer is: a) SEQOHS accreditation is a UK voluntary requirement

SEQOHS accreditation is a UK-based voluntary scheme. It is not a legal requirement but is used by employers and occupational health services in the UK to demonstrate adherence to high standards of practice.

Source: www.fom.ac.uk/media-events/publications/seqohs-publications

QUESTION 21

You are reviewing the skin surveillance system for a large hairdressing chain. All employees have completed a baseline high-level health surveillance questionnaire and visual inspection, but follow-up surveillance has not been conducted for two years.

When should the follow-up surveillance have been conducted for these employees?

The answer is: a) At 6 weeks, 12 weeks, and then annually

According to HSE guidelines for high-level skin surveillance, after the baseline assessment, employees should have had follow-up assessments at 6 weeks and 12 weeks.

HSE guidance outlines the requirements for skin surveillance in workplaces where there is potential exposure to harmful agents.

High-level skin surveillance is required when employees are exposed to high-risk agents with the potential to cause harm through skin contact. It involves a structured schedule of questionnaires and skin examinations:
- Baseline assessment (before first exposure)
- Week 6 (after starting exposure)

- Week 12
- Annually thereafter.

If a skin problem is reported, it must be followed up with a visual skin examination and proper documentation.

Low-level skin surveillance is suitable when:
- direct skin contact is usually avoided
- exposure control is adequate
- there is only occasional or potential exposure
- there is only suggestive evidence of a hazard.

In low-level surveillance, after a baseline assessment, employees complete an annual questionnaire. If symptoms are reported, they undergo a skin examination, and the frequency of surveillance may be increased along with a review of risk assessments and control measures.

Source: www.som.org.uk/sites/som.org.uk/files/SOM_Managing_Skin_Health_at_Work_Nov_2023.pdf

QUESTION 22

You see a 29-year-old warehouse operator with non-specific upper limb pain who has been absent from work for 4 weeks.

What is the best intervention to help him to return to work?

The answer is: c) Multidisciplinary rehabilitation including both physical and psychosocial approaches

The summary of recommendations for workers with non-specific arm pain and tenosynovitis includes the following for workers with non-specific arm pain absent for at least four weeks:
- Employers should offer or facilitate multidisciplinary rehabilitation programmes that include both physical and psychosocial approaches
- Physical sessions should be led by a health professional (e.g. physiotherapist or occupational therapist) focusing on strength, endurance, relaxation, energy conservation and ergonomics education
- Psychosocial sessions should be led by a health professional (e.g. psychologist or occupational therapist) using cognitive behavioural techniques to improve coping strategies and prepare for return to work

Answers to Mock exam 2

- An individualised return-to-work plan should be agreed upon in advance, involving the rehabilitation team, employer and worker
- Employers should consider temporarily modifying duties for workers whose condition is aggravated by work.

Source: www.rcp.ac.uk/media/iajpo4ke/upper-limb-disorders-national-guideline.pdf

QUESTION 23

You are an occupational health specialist conducting a workplace visit at a farm where employees regularly handle various farm animals. During your visit, you discuss zoonotic diseases and workplace safety with the farm manager.

Which one of the following legislations specifically applies to the risk assessment of zoonoses and their control measures in the workplace?

The answer is: a) COSHH (Control of Substances Hazardous to Health Regulations) 2002

COSHH (Control of Substances Hazardous to Health Regulations) 2002: this regulation specifically applies to the risk assessment and control of hazardous substances in the workplace, including biological agents such as zoonotic pathogens. It requires employers to assess risks, implement control measures and maintain safety standards for handling such substances, making it directly relevant to managing zoonoses.

HASAWA (Health and Safety at Work etc. Act) 1974: while this act provides the overall framework for health and safety in the workplace, including risk assessments, it does not specifically target the control of biological hazards such as zoonoses. It covers general duties of employers and employees but is not as specific as COSHH in addressing hazardous substances.

Management of Health and Safety at Work Regulations 1999: these regulations require employers to conduct risk assessments and implement health and safety measures. However, they are broader in scope and do not specifically address the control of biological agents or zoonoses, which is the domain of COSHH.

Public Health (Control of Disease) Act 1984: this Act focuses on public health measures and disease control at the community level rather than workplace-specific regulations. It is concerned with the broader management of disease outbreaks rather than individual workplace risk assessments.

Health Protection (Notification) Regulations 2010: these regulations are concerned with the notification of certain diseases and the protection of public health. They do not specifically address the workplace risk assessment and control measures for zoonoses, which are covered under COSHH.

Source: www.hse.gov.uk/agriculture/topics/zoonoses.htm

QUESTION 24

During a training session for healthcare professionals you are discussing the importance of safeguarding patient information. A colleague asks about the purpose of the Caldicott Principles and their relevance to sharing information within health and social care settings.

Which of the following best describes the primary purpose of the Caldicott Principles?

The answer is: b) To inform good information sharing while protecting the confidentiality of patient records

The Caldicott Principles provide a framework for good information sharing while protecting the confidentiality of patient records to support safe and effective care.

They consist of eight principles designed to ensure the appropriate and secure use of confidential information in health and social care. They aim to balance confidentiality with the necessity of information sharing for safe and effective care, including purposes beyond individual care, such as public interest. These principles apply to all identifiable data collected for health and social care and sometimes staff information, emphasising transparency and patient involvement.

The eight principles:
1. Justify the purpose for using confidential information, ensuring it is necessary and regularly reviewed.
2. Use confidential information only when necessary for the intended purpose.
3. Use the minimum necessary information required for the task.
4. Restrict access on a need-to-know basis to those who require it.
5. Ensure all with access understand their responsibilities to maintain confidentiality.
6. Comply with the law, ensuring lawful use of confidential information.

Answers to Mock exam 2

7. Balance the duty to share information for care with the duty to protect confidentiality.
8. Inform patients and service users about how their information is used and their choices.

They do not alter the principle that Occupational Health records must not be shared outside of OH without consent.

While the principles encourage information sharing to support care, they emphasise protecting confidentiality, not unrestricted sharing.

The Caldicott Principles balance the need for effective information sharing with the obligation to safeguard confidentiality, ensuring safe and appropriate use of patient data.

The principles are ethical guidelines, not a legal framework.

The principles stress the importance of both sharing and protecting information to enable care.

Consent is not required in all cases, such as when sharing is necessary for direct care under professional duty.

Source: www.ukcgc.uk/the-caldicott-principles

QUESTION 25

You are assessing a 50-year-old gardener who shows you photos of a linear rash on sun-exposed areas of their skin. The rash has led to significant post-inflammatory pigmentation where the marks previously were. The management team are seeking advice on managing their condition.

What is the most likely diagnosis?

The answer is: e) Phytophotodermatitis

Phytophotodermatitis ("strimmer's dermatitis") is a skin condition that occurs when photosensitive plant chemicals come into contact with the skin and then are exposed to sunlight (UV light). This results in a characteristic linear rash and significant post-inflammatory pigmentation in the affected areas. This fits the description of the gardener's condition where the rash is localised to sun-exposed areas and exhibits post-inflammatory pigmentation.

Allergic contact dermatitis to plants: usually presents as an itchy rash and may not have a linear pattern or post-inflammatory pigmentation.

Burns: would typically cause immediate damage and are less likely to have a linear appearance based on plant exposure.

Non-accidental injury: would be considered if the cause of the rash was unclear, but the pattern and pigmentation suggest a different aetiology.

Dermatitis artefacta: involves self-induced dermatitis often related to psychological factors, not typically presenting with a linear rash from plant exposure.

Source: https://dermnetnz.org/topics/phytophotodermatitis

QUESTION 26

A 36-year-old employee has been managing long-term depression with counselling, which allows her to perform normal day-to-day activities effectively. Her employer seeks advice on whether the Equality Act 2010 is likely to apply in this case.

Under the Equality Act 2010, how should the impact of the employee's depression best be assessed to determine if it qualifies as a disability?

The answer is: d) The effect of treatment is disregarded when assessing whether the condition has a substantial adverse effect on day-to-day activities

Under the Equality Act 2010, when determining whether a person has a disability, the effect of any treatment or correction is disregarded. This means that the individual's condition should be assessed as if the treatment (in this case, counselling) was not in place. If the depression would have a substantial adverse effect on the employee's ability to carry out normal day-to-day activities without treatment for a duration of 12 months or more, the condition would likely qualify as a disability under the Act.

While the duration of the condition is relevant, the key issue in this scenario is whether the treatment's effect is disregarded when assessing the impact on day-to-day activities.

Source: https://assets.publishing.service.gov.uk/media/5a80dcc8ed915d74e6230df4/Equality_Act_2010-disability_definition.pdf

QUESTION 27

You are involved in setting up a health surveillance programme for vibration exposure in a construction company about to commence operations. The company has a tight budget and wants to know who the most cost-effective person might be to administer tier 2 questionnaires.

What is the most appropriate option?

The answer is: a) A responsible person

Employers can appoint a responsible person to carry out the simple screening using the Tier 2 questionnaire as part of the health surveillance programme. This is likely to be the most appropriate choice as it is compliant and cost-effective.

This can be any employee as part of their role.

This person:
- should be carefully selected to have experience of the working environment and be able to gain the confidence and cooperation of employees
- need not be qualified but should have received training from an occupational health professional
- should understand the health surveillance procedures, the process of referral to an occupational health professional (e.g. following a positive questionnaire response), and the need to treat information confidentially
- should be able to describe to the employee the symptoms of HAVS but should not attempt to diagnose disease
- should not make judgements about the cause of the symptoms if an employee discloses that they have symptoms.

Sources:
- www.som.org.uk/sites/som.org.uk/files/HAVS_Guidance_from_SOM_v16.pdf
- www.bali.org.uk/help-and-advice/documents/health-surveillance-for-hand-arm-vibration-syndrome/health-surveillance-for-hand-arm-vibration-syndrome.pdf

QUESTION 28

You are an occupational health physician remotely assessing a 50-year-old receptionist who recently underwent an uncomplicated total abdominal hysterectomy. She is eager to return to work and her employer seeks advice on when it might be appropriate to do so.

Based on current guidelines, when are most women able to return to work after an uncomplicated total abdominal hysterectomy?

The answer is: b) Most women are able to return to work by 6–8 weeks after an uncomplicated abdominal hysterectomy, depending on their recovery

Current guidelines suggest that most women can return to work within 6 to 8 weeks following an uncomplicated abdominal hysterectomy, although the specific timing depends on the individual's recovery and the nature of their job.

Source: www.rcog.org.uk/for-the-public/browse-our-patient-information/abdominal-hysterectomy-recovering-well

QUESTION 29

You are undertaking a workplace visit to a bottling plant.

You undertake a one-off noise reading as you have found it to be very noisy.

The reading is 98 dB(A).

Workers are not wearing any PPE and there are no signs to indicate that this is a restricted area.

What is the most appropriate next step?

The answer is: b) Advise a formal noise survey

Further investigation of a one-off reading is needed to determine each worker's daily or weekly personal noise exposure (LEP,d or LEP,w) to assess what further action is needed under the Control of Noise at Work Regulations 2005.

The daily personal noise exposure (LEP,d) is the time-averaged, A-weighted noise level for a nominal 8-hour working day, used for assessing the noise exposure of a worker during a working day. If the noise exposure of workers varies markedly from day to day, the personal noise exposure may also be assessed over a week rather than a day and is noted as the LEP,w.

QUESTION 30

You see a pregnant employee with a complicated pregnancy. She enquires about her rights regarding time off for antenatal (pregnancy-related) appointments.

Which one of the following statements about time off for antenatal appointments is correct?

The answer is: b) Pregnant employees are entitled to paid time off for antenatal appointments

Pregnant employees are legally entitled to paid time off for antenatal appointments, which covers medical appointments related to pregnancy, as well as classes for health, fitness and relaxation, and sessions that support mental health and wellbeing. This paid time off also includes travel time. While there is no strict limit on the number of appointments, the law specifies a 'reasonable' amount, typically up to 10 appointments for a first baby and around 7 for subsequent pregnancies. Employers can request evidence of the appointments after the first one.

Source: www.acas.org.uk/managing-your-employees-maternity-leave-and-pay/attending-pregnancy-related-appointments

QUESTION 31

You are conducting a training session for Diploma students on workplace safety. During the session, you explain the importance of conducting risk assessments to identify potential hazards. One of the employees asks how risk is calculated in the context of a risk assessment and risk matrices.

Which of the following best describes how risk is calculated?

The answer is: c) Risk = Likelihood × Severity

In risk assessments, risk is typically calculated by multiplying the likelihood (or probability) of an event occurring by the severity of the consequences if the event occurs. This approach helps in quantifying risk and prioritising which hazards need more urgent control measures.

While 'impact' is similar to 'severity', the correct term used in the standard risk formula is 'severity'. Additionally, the term 'likelihood' (or probability) is used rather than 'frequency' in standard risk assessment calculations.

QUESTION 32

You are an occupational health doctor conducting a health assessment for Mr Patel, a 40-year-old worker in the construction industry. He has been exposed to respirable crystalline silica (RCS) for 15 years. You review his respiratory questionnaire and lung function tests, which are unremarkable.

What further investigation does Mr Patel most require as part of health surveillance for silica exposure?

The answer is: a) Chest X-ray

Guidelines recommend a PA chest X-ray after 15 years of RCS exposure and subsequently every 3 years thereafter. This routine screening helps in early detection of lung abnormalities associated with silica exposure.

A Covid test is used to diagnose acute infection with the SARS-CoV-2 virus causing Covid-19. It is not relevant to monitoring silica exposure-related lung diseases such as silicosis, which develop over years of exposure to silica dust and are unrelated to viral infections.

CT scans are more sensitive than chest X-rays in detecting subtle lung abnormalities. However, they are typically reserved for cases where chest X-rays show abnormalities or when there is a high clinical suspicion of lung disease beyond what X-rays can detect. Routine use of CT scans for surveillance purposes in silica-exposed individuals without specific indications is not supported by current guidelines, due to radiation exposure and cost considerations.

The Mantoux test, also known as the tuberculin skin test, is used to detect tuberculosis (TB) infection. It is not part of the health surveillance monitoring of silica.

Source: www.hse.gov.uk/pubns/priced/healthsurveillance.pdf

QUESTION 33

You see a new receptionist in the radiology department who is worried about the risk of cancer from radiation exposure.

Which of the following is the most appropriate for the effect she is describing?

The answer is: e) Stochastic effect

Stochastic effects are those that occur by chance and do not have a threshold dose, with the probability of occurrence increasing with dose. Cancer is a classic example of a stochastic effect. This term precisely describes the type of risk the receptionist is worried about, making it the most correct and appropriate answer.

Deterministic effects, also known as non-stochastic effects, are those health effects that increase in severity with higher doses of radiation and have a threshold below which they do not occur. Examples of deterministic effects are skin erythema and hair loss.

Hereditary effects refer to genetic mutations that can be passed on to offspring because of radiation exposure. While important, the receptionist's concern is about her own risk of developing cancer, not about potential genetic effects on her future children.

Late-onset effect: while cancer can indeed be a late-onset effect, this term is less precise and less commonly used in the context of radiation risks. Thus, it is not the most accurate description of the receptionist's concern.

Random effect is a very general term and does not specifically pertain to the nature of radiation-induced cancer. While cancer risk from radiation exposure does involve random mutations at the cellular level, the term 'random effect' lacks the specificity needed to accurately describe this risk, making it less correct than other options.

QUESTION 34

You are conducting a workplace visit to a bakery that is monitoring the flour concentration as part of their risk monitoring process. The exposure is measured over two key time periods: long-term and short-term.

What are the two time periods used to measure workplace exposure limits (WELs) in the UK?

The answer is: c) 8 hours (long-term) and 15 minutes (short-term)

WELs are UK occupational exposure limits (OELs) designed to protect workers' health by specifying allowable concentrations of hazardous substances in the air. These limits are measured as time-weighted averages (TWA) over two periods: long-term (8 hours) and short-term (15 minutes). Short-term exposure limits (STELs) are particularly used to prevent acute effects, such as irritation, from brief exposures.

QUESTION 35

You are evaluating a study that examines the mortality rates among workers exposed to a specific occupational hazard. In this study, the researchers use the general population as a comparison group to mortality. The results show that the workers have a lower observed mortality risk compared to the general population.

What type of bias may be having the most influence on the study's findings?

The answer is: d) Healthy worker effect

In cohort studies that compare mortality in an occupational group with that in the general population, bias may arise from a 'healthy worker effect'. This occurs because employed people tend on average to be healthier than the population at large. In particular, people with chronic disabling disease have the potential to be selectively excluded from employment. Thus, when followed up over time, employed populations tend to have lower than average death rates.

Source: Sadhra, S., Bray, A.J. and Boorman, S. (eds) (2022) *Oxford Handbook of Occupational Health*, 3rd edition

QUESTION 36

You see Mx Jessop, a 45-year-old employee with substance misuse concerns. The employee disagrees with your opinion that they are fit to return to work with adjustments. Subsequently, the employer calls you after receiving a message from your administrator that they will not receive a report as the employee has withdrawn consent. The manager explains that she has paid for the report and is unable to further manage the employee's erratic absences without it.

What is the most appropriate course of action for you to take in this situation?

The answer is: d) Explain to the employer that no further information can be disclosed without the employee's consent

According to General Medical Council (GMC) guidance, patient confidentiality is paramount. Information cannot be shared without the explicit consent of the patient. The Faculty of Occupational Medicine (FOM) also emphasises the need for informed consent before disclosing any medical information to employers. This option respects the legal and ethical requirement to maintain patient confidentiality.

Discussing the reasons for withdrawal of consent would still involve disclosing personal information without the employee's consent. This breaches confidentiality and is not permissible under GMC and FOM guidelines.

Sending a summary of a report without consent violates the principle of confidentiality. Any report or summary sent without the patient's consent is a breach of trust and against GMC and FOM guidelines.

While advising the employer to contact the employee directly respects the confidentiality principle, it places undue pressure on the employee and could be seen as the employer trying to circumvent the need for consent. The appropriate approach is to inform the employer that they cannot receive the information without consent, not to suggest alternative means of obtaining it.

While option b) (Explain that the employer needs to manage the case with the information that they already have) might be practically helpful to the employer, it does not address the core issue of confidentiality and consent directly.
The primary focus should be on the legal and ethical inability to provide further information without consent, rather than on how the employer should proceed with existing information.

Sources:
- Sadhra, S., Bray, A.J. and Boorman, S. (eds) (2022) *Oxford Handbook of Occupational Health*, 3rd edition
- www.fom.ac.uk/wp-content/uploads/conffomoct09kloss.pdf
- www.gmc-uk.org/professional-standards/professional-standards-for-doctors/decision-making-and-consent

QUESTION 37

A 65-year-old construction worker presents with concerns about progressive contracture of his fingers. On examination, you observe thickening and shortening of the palmar fascia with noticeable contracture in his fingers.

Which of the following statements about Dupuytren's disease (DD) is most accurate?

The answer is: b) Dupuytren's disease is associated with conditions such as diabetes

Dupuytren's disease (DD) is known to be more prevalent in men and its incidence increases with age. The condition is consistently associated with health conditions such as diabetes, liver disease and epilepsy, and there is a significant genetic component influencing its development. It is also linked to vibration exposure. The prevalence of DD increases with age, making option b) the most accurate statement regarding the disease.

Source: www.som.org.uk/sites/som.org.uk/files/Dupuytrens_Disease_and_work_with_hand-held_vibrating_tools.pdf

QUESTION 38

You are an occupational health advisor at a medium-sized manufacturing company. An employee has been on sick leave due to illness, and approaches you to discuss the company's policy on providing documentation for their absence. They are unsure about the requirements after being off work for more than a week.

Which one of the following would be the most appropriate for you to inform the employee regarding the requirement for a 'fit note' (sick note)?

The answer is: b) A 'fit note' is required if the employee has been ill and off work for more than 7 consecutive days

Employees must provide their employer with a 'fit note' (also known as a 'sick note') if they have been ill and on sick leave for more than 7 consecutive days. This requirement includes non-working days such as weekends and bank holidays. This documentation helps the employer understand the duration and nature of the employee's illness and plan for any necessary adjustments or support.

Source: www.gov.uk/taking-sick-leave

QUESTION 39

At a bustling construction site a team is focused on concrete cutting and drilling operations on the ground floor.

The construction manager, concerned about the potential health hazards posed by airborne dust generated during these activities, has implemented a wet spray dust suppression system.

Which term best describes this type of control?

The answer is: c) Engineering

Water spray systems are designed to apply water to the cutting or grinding surface to wet the surface and prevent the resulting dust from becoming airborne. Many construction tools/equipment types can be purchased with wet spray attachments. Water can also be manually applied to the concrete surface before and during the work (grinding, drilling, cutting, etc.). This is a form of engineering control.

The Hierarchy of Control outlines progressive steps for managing health and safety risks in the workplace, aiming to reduce hazards to as low as reasonably practicable:

Elimination: this is the most effective control measure where hazards are completely removed from the workplace. This can be achieved by redesigning processes, substituting hazardous materials with safer alternatives, or adopting alternative methods that eliminate the need for hazardous tasks.

Substitution: when elimination is not possible, substitution involves replacing hazardous substances, equipment, or processes with less hazardous alternatives. This approach minimises risks by introducing safer elements into the workplace, such as using non-toxic chemicals or safer equipment.

Engineering controls: such controls focus on isolating workers from hazards through physical modifications in the workplace. This includes installing barriers, improving ventilation systems, or introducing automated machinery to reduce exposure to risks.

Administrative controls: these modify work practices, procedures or policies to reduce risks. Examples include providing training on hazard awareness, rotating employees through tasks, or limiting access to hazardous areas. While not as effective as eliminating or substituting hazards, administrative controls are crucial in managing risks.

Personal protective equipment: PPE is the last line of defence and includes equipment such as helmets, gloves and masks. It should be used when other controls are not sufficient. Employers must ensure proper selection, training, maintenance and compliance with PPE to protect workers effectively.

QUESTION 40

You are the occupational health advisor for a company that employs several night shift workers. The management team is reviewing its policies regarding health assessments for night workers. One of the managers asks you if employees are required to undergo health assessments before starting night work.

Which of the following is the most accurate response regarding the requirement for night workers to undergo health assessments?

The answer is: c) Night workers must be offered a health assessment before starting night work, but they are not obligated to accept it

Employers must offer a health assessment before night work begins, but workers are not legally required to accept it. They have the option to decline.

The requirement to offer health assessments applies to all night workers in the UK, not just in England.

There is no requirement for attendance at follow-up assessments.

Source: www.gov.uk/night-working-hours/health-assessments

QUESTION 41

During a workplace visit to a film studio, you notice that the general lighting appears poor.

Which one of the following potential costs to the business is most likely to result from inadequate lighting?

The answer is: e) All of the above

Poor lighting can lead to multiple costs for a business, including the following:
- *Time off work because of accidents and injuries*: inadequate lighting increases the likelihood of accidents and injuries, leading to employees taking time off work
- *Increased absenteeism*: poor lighting can cause discomfort or strain, potentially leading to higher rates of absenteeism
- *Reduced staff efficiency*: insufficient lighting can hinder employees' ability to see clearly and perform tasks efficiently
- *Reduced productivity*: poor lighting can affect workers' performance and productivity, as they may struggle to complete their tasks effectively.

Therefore, all these factors can be significant costs associated with poor lighting in the workplace.

Source: www.hse.gov.uk/pubns/priced/hsg38.pdf

QUESTION 42

You see an individual with long Covid who has been absent from work for 6 months. The employer would like advice on the likelihood of return to work.

Based on general guidance, what is estimated likelihood of return to work?

The answer is: e) 50%

The FOM provides guidance for healthcare professionals on helping patients with post-Covid syndrome return to work.

Key points include:
- Work benefits health by providing purpose and financial independence
- Prolonged worklessness can lead to poor physical and mental health, increasing the risk of self-harm
- The likelihood of not returning to work rises the longer a person is off sick
- After six months of sick leave, the chance of returning to work is approximately 50%
- Returning to work is crucial for rehabilitation from various illnesses and important for overall health.

Source: www.fom.ac.uk/wp-content/uploads/FOM-Guidance-post-COVID_healthcare-professionals.pdf

QUESTION 43

You are teaching an occupational health trainee about safety-critical tasks.

Which of the following best defines a safety-critical task?

The answer is: c) A task where personal impairment or error can jeopardise the safety of others or lead to a critical incident

A task where personal impairment or error can jeopardise the safety of others or lead to a critical incident: this definition captures the essence of a safety-critical task, where personal impairment can affect the safety of others or result in significant incidents.

Another way of defining safety-critical work is any task that (in the event of failure) may lead to an accident, or otherwise compromise the safety of:
- people (employees, clients or service users, the public)
- plant or premises
- the environment.

Sources:
- Hobson, J. and Smedley, J. (eds) (2019) *Fitness for Work: the medical aspects*, 6th edition. Oxford University Press
- Sadhra, S., Bray, A.J. and Boorman, S. (eds) (2022) *Oxford Handbook of Occupational Health*, 3rd edition

QUESTION 44

You are planning a health promotion session for construction workers. You have been asked to focus on the main occupational health risks of construction work.

According to the HSE, what is the main risk to health that construction workers encounter?

The answer is: a) Asbestos

According to the Health and Safety Executive (HSE), asbestos remains the biggest occupational health risk to construction workers. Inhalation of asbestos fibres can cause mesothelioma, lung cancer and asbestosis. Asbestos is commonly found in older buildings, making it crucial for workers to take proper precautions when handling or disturbing materials that may contain it.

Silica is the second biggest risk to construction workers.

Source: www.hse.gov.uk/construction/healthrisks/cancer-and-construction/asbestos.htm

QUESTION 45

You are an occupational health professional assessing the potential health effects of whole body vibration (WBV) on a group of heavy machinery operators.

Which of the following health effects is most commonly associated with WBV exposure?

The answer is: d) Increased risk of lumbar spine disease

The primary risk is of low back pain (LBP), which may be non-specific or resulting from lumbar disc degeneration.

Other suggested effects including hypertension, neck pain and cervical disc degeneration, autonomic disturbance, and digestive and reproductive effects

Answers to Mock exam 2

are less well evidenced. Motion sickness and *mal de debarquement* syndrome are well recognised.

Sources:
- www.som.org.uk/sites/som.org.uk/files/HAVS_and_Whole_Body_Vibration_Feb_2023.pdf
- Sadhra, S., Bray, A.J. and Boorman, S. (eds) (2022) *Oxford Handbook of Occupational Health*, 3rd edition

QUESTION 46

During a workplace visit to a construction site with 100 employees, you request to see the accident book, but the employer does not have one.

What is the most appropriate action regarding the employer's legal obligations?

The answer is: c) Advise the employer that they must purchase or create an accident book as required by law and keep it to record all workplace incidents

Employers with more than ten employees are legally required to maintain an accident book to record all workplace incidents. This requirement is mandatory and not contingent on requests from insurance companies or inspections by the HSE. The legal obligation specifies that a record system must be in place to document accidents and injuries to comply with this legal requirement and ensure proper documentation and risk management.

Source: www.hse.gov.uk/simple-health-safety/reporting-accidents-ill-health.htm

QUESTION 47

You are conducting a workplace visit at a construction site where cement is being used extensively. During the visit, you notice a worker kneeling in wet cement without proper protective gear. The worker appears unaware of the potential dangers associated with wet cement exposure.

Which option best describes the occupational health risks of exposure to wet cement?

The answer is: e) All of the above

Wet cement poses multiple occupational health risks due to its high alkalinity and the presence of sensitising agents such as hexavalent chromium. The risks include:
- Skin burns: wet cement can cause chemical burns due to its alkalinity, especially if it is trapped against the skin
- Allergic dermatitis: repeated exposure to wet cement can lead to allergic contact dermatitis due to the presence of sensitisers
- Irritant dermatitis: wet cement can cause irritant contact dermatitis as a result of its caustic nature
- Ocular chemical burns: splashes of wet cement can cause severe chemical burns to the eyes, potentially leading to permanent damage.

Therefore, all the options listed are valid health risks associated with wet cement exposure, emphasising the need for proper controls and awareness among workers.

Source: www.hse.gov.uk/pubns/cis26.pdf

QUESTION 48

During a routine health assessment, you discover that an employee, who operates heavy machinery, has developed a severe health condition that could impair their ability to work safely. The employee insists that you do not disclose this information to their employer due to fear of losing their job. You are aware that disclosing this information could prevent potential harm to other employees and the public.

What are the most important aspects to consider when deciding whether to disclose this information in the public interest?

The answer is: b) The severity and nature of the health condition and the risk it poses to others

The GMC advises that, in situations where there is a need to disclose information in the public interest, several factors should be considered. These include the nature of the information to be disclosed, what use will be made of it, the number of people who will receive the information, the safeguards in place to protect the information, and the potential for distress or harm to patients. The overriding need for disclosure in the interests of public safety is particularly important. The occupational physician should consider the risk posed by the employee's health condition to the safety of others and seek advice from colleagues or a professional body if unsure.

While patient consent and fears are important, they are not the primary concern when public safety is at risk.

Legal implications are a consideration but are not the primary factor when determining the public interest disclosure.

Source: www.fom.ac.uk/wp-content/uploads/GOMP_2017_Web.pdf

QUESTION 49

A 34-year-old woman, who is applying for a promotion, discloses to her manager that she had severe depression when she was 18. The condition had a substantial and long-term adverse effect on her ability to carry out normal day-to-day activities at the time, but she has fully recovered and has not experienced any recurrence. The employer expresses concern about her past mental illness and is hesitant to promote her based on this information.

Under the Equality Act 2010, which one of the following statements is true regarding her protection against discrimination in this situation?

The answer is: b) She is protected under the Act as a person with a past disability

The Equality Act 2010 provides protection for individuals who have had a disability in the past, even if they have fully recovered. They will be protected by the Act if discriminated against because of the past disability.

The Act's protection does not depend on the recurrence of the condition. The protection is not contingent on when or if the condition was disclosed.

The Act does not impose a time limit on how recent the condition must have been to qualify for protection.

Source: https://assets.publishing.service.gov.uk/media/5a80dcc8ed915d74e6230df4/Equality_Act_2010-disability_definition.pdf

QUESTION 50

A 30-year-old worker with epilepsy accepts a job offer to operate heavy machinery in a manufacturing plant. The job involves working around unguarded moving parts and heights, where sudden loss of consciousness could result in serious injury. The worker does not disclose their medical condition to the employer during the pre-employment process. After a few weeks on the job, the worker has a seizure and is injured. An investigation into the incident raises concerns about whether the employee fulfilled their legal obligations under health and safety law.

Under the Health and Safety at Work etc. Act 1974 (HASAWA), which of the following statements best describes the employee's duties related to health and safety?

The answer is: c) The employee has a duty to take reasonable care of their own health and safety, which includes disclosing relevant medical conditions that could pose a hazard

Employees are obligated under the Health and Safety at Work etc. Act 1974 (HASAWA) to "take reasonable care" for their own health and safety, as well as that of others. This includes cooperating on health and safety matters and avoiding actions that could jeopardise their own safety or that of others. This duty may extend to the disclosure of relevant medical conditions after a job offer has been made. For instance, if an employee does not disclose that they have epilepsy before beginning a job where this could present a hazard, they might be in violation of their responsibilities under Section 7 of HASAWA.

Source: Hobson, J. and Smedley, J. (eds) (2019) *Fitness for Work: the medical aspects*, 6th edition. Oxford University Press

QUESTION 51

You review the blood lead levels for a 25-year-old woman. They are 25 µg/dl.

Reference values:

Action level – a blood lead concentration of:
- 25 µg/dl in a woman of reproductive capacity
- 40 µg/dl in a young person
- 50 µg/dl in any other employee

Suspension level – a blood lead concentration of:
- 30 µg/dl in a woman of reproductive capacity
- 50 µg/dl in a young person
- 60 µg/dl in any other employee

Answers to Mock exam 2

What should you advise the employer to be the most appropriate next step?

The answer is: a) Carry out an urgent investigation to find out why this has happened

The next step is an urgent investigation. It is crucial to determine the source of lead exposure and review the efficacy of control measures. Identifying the cause is the first step in preventing further exposure and protecting the health of the employee and others who might be at risk. The aim is to prevent the worker's blood lead level reaching the suspension level. Improvements or changes might be required to ensure adequate protection.

Action levels: these are concentrations of lead in blood set below the threshold for suspension. If these levels are reached or exceeded, the employer must:
- conduct an urgent investigation to determine the cause;
- review existing control measures; and
- take feasible steps to reduce the employee's blood lead concentration below the action level.

Suspension levels: these are concentrations of lead in blood or urine that typically result in employees being temporarily removed from lead-exposed work, to prevent the risk of lead poisoning.

Source: www.hse.gov.uk/pubns/priced/l132.pdf

QUESTION 52

You encounter a 35-year-old baker presenting with symptoms suggestive of occupational asthma. Spirometry reveals an obstructive pattern.

Which is the most appropriate investigation to establish a diagnosis?

The answer is: c) Serial peak flows

The first-line diagnostic tests for occupational asthma (OA) should ideally be conducted early, prior to starting maintenance therapy, and while the patient is still exposed to potential allergens at work.

Serial peak expiratory flow (PEF) recordings are the next line of investigation.

Other relevant tests to aid making a diagnosis include:
- Immunological testing: specific IgE and skin prick tests (SPT)
- Non-specific bronchial hyper-responsiveness (NSBHR) testing
- Bronchial provocation challenge.

Source: www.brit-thoracic.org.uk/quality-improvement/clinical-statements/occupational-asthma

QUESTION 53

You see a 40-year-old psychiatry registrar who is currently 30 weeks pregnant. She works in a sedentary role with minimal manual handling and works up to 50 hours a week. As part of her revised pregnancy risk assessment, her employer wishes to reduce her working hours. The employee wishes to continue working as usual until she starts her maternity leave.

What is the most appropriate advice to give her employer?

The answer is: c) She can continue to work long hours if she wishes, with an understanding of the risks

The RCP publication *Physical and Shift Work in Pregnancy: occupational aspects of management* states the following:

- Employers must conduct a risk assessment when informed of an employee's pregnancy. This assessment should consider physical demands and duration of tasks.
- Heavy physical work and lifting are moderately risky for low birth weight and intrauterine growth restriction (IUGR). Employers should reduce very heavy physical activities and lifting, especially in late pregnancy, but restrictions should not be imposed if the pregnant worker chooses to continue.
- Standing for more than 3 hours has a small risk of preterm birth and low birth weight. Employers should reduce prolonged standing in late pregnancy but should respect the worker's choice to continue if informed of the risks.
- Long working hours pose a small to moderate risk of preterm birth and low birth weight. Working hours should be limited to about 40 per week in late pregnancy if possible, but restrictions should not be imposed if the worker chooses to continue.
- There is insufficient evidence to recommend restricting shift work, including rotating shifts or night work.

Therefore, while it is advisable to reduce working hours to about 40 per week in late pregnancy to mitigate risks, this recommendation should be balanced with the worker's wishes. Since the worker wants to continue as normal, this option is not the most appropriate.

The Equality Act protects against discrimination but does not give an absolute right to work in any condition. Employers still have a duty to ensure a safe working environment. Therefore, this option is not fully accurate.

Redeployment is unnecessary unless there are specific risks that cannot be mitigated in her current role. The worker wishes to continue her current role, so this option is not appropriate.

Source: www.nhshealthatwork.co.uk/images/library/files/Clinical%20excellence/Pregnancy-FullGuidelines.pdf

QUESTION 54

You are working with the safety team who have performed a risk assessment requiring the use of half mask respirators in environments with silica dust.

What is the most appropriate next step the employer should take to ensure optimal control is provided when implementing this change?

The answer is: c) Fit test

To ensure adequate protection all tight-fitting respiratory protection equipment (RPE) must be fit tested as part of the initial selection stage. Fit testing checks that the mask forms a proper seal on the individual's face, preventing silica dust from leaking in and being inhaled. Without a proper fit, the respirator may not be effective, leaving workers at risk of exposure to harmful silica dust.

While other steps such as providing information on how to use the mask, ensuring appropriate storage, conducting health surveillance, and dust monitoring are also important, the initial priority should be to ensure that the respirators fit properly and provide effective protection.

Health surveillance is an important ongoing measure to monitor workers for any signs of adverse health effects due to exposure to silica dust. This can help in early detection of issues and timely intervention. However, it is a follow-up step that should be conducted after ensuring that the respiratory protective equipment is effectively preventing exposure, starting with a fit test.

Ensuring appropriate storage of respirators is important to maintain their integrity and functionality. Proper storage prevents damage and contamination, ensuring that the respirators remain effective over time. While this is necessary for long-term maintenance, it does not directly address the immediate need to verify that the respirators provide adequate protection through a fit test.

Dust monitoring is crucial for assessing the levels of silica dust in the work environment and ensuring that control measures are effective. It helps in verifying that exposure levels are within safe limits and can inform the need for further controls. However, before performing dust monitoring, it is imperative to ensure that the respirators provide effective protection through a fit test, making fit testing the more immediate priority to optimise the control measures.

Providing information on how to use the mask is essential for ensuring that workers understand how to correctly wear and maintain their respirators. This includes guidance on how to don and doff the mask, check for a proper seal each time it is worn, and perform routine maintenance. However, this step should follow the fit test to ensure that the respirators being used are effective for each individual. Training on usage is critical but is not the immediate next step before ensuring a proper fit.

Sources:
- https://books.hse.gov.uk/gempdf/hsg53.pdf
- Sadhra, S., Bray, A.J. and Boorman, S. (eds) (2022) *Oxford Handbook of Occupational Health*, 3rd edition

QUESTION 55

You are visiting a farm on a workplace visit. When talking to a sheep farmer, you notice a lesion on her finger. She tells you that this started as a reddish-blue lump which enlarged to a flat-topped, blood-tinged pustule about 2–3 cm across. She says it is painless.

What is the most likely diagnosis?

The answer is: e) Orf

Orf is a common skin disease caused by a parapox virus affecting sheep and goats, which can spread to humans in close contact with infected animals. It causes localised skin lesions and is not serious.

It causes pustular or scabby lesions around the mouth and nostrils of lambs, which may spread to the teats of ewes and the legs of lambs. It is transmitted to humans through direct contact with infected animals.

Occupations and processes at risk:
- *Contact with infected animals*: activities such as bottle-feeding lambs, sheep shearing and slaughtering sheep

- *Handling materials from infected animals*: particularly handling infected wool or carcasses
- *Contact with recently vaccinated animals or vaccine injuries*: risk of infection through close contact or inoculation injuries.

Source: www.nhs.uk/conditions/orf

QUESTION 56

Reported cases of toxoplasmosis in the UK are fairly rare. However, it is estimated that up to a third of the population are infected with *Toxoplasma gondii* at some time in their lives.

From the list below, which animal is most likely to spread this infection?

The answer is: b) Cats

Cats are the most common source of the *Toxoplasma* protozoa that are transmitted to other animals or people.

The main routes of spread are the ingestion of water, food or soil contaminated with faeces from infected cats, or the consumption of undercooked meat (mainly pork or lamb). The parasite can also be spread from infected sheep at lambing time.

Occupational exposure to *Toxoplasma gondii* may occur in those who:
- are in contact with infected cats or cat faeces;
- are in contact with infected sheep during lambing; or
- work with materials or products from infected animals.

Sources:
- www.nhs.uk/conditions/toxoplasmosis
- www.hse.ie/eng/services/list/5/publichealth/publichealthdepts/pub/toxo-leaflet.pdf
- www.hpsc.ie/a-z/zoonotic/toxoplasmosis/factsheets

QUESTION 57

During a workplace visit in an office, you notice that it is quite cold even on a summer's day, and many employees are still wearing their coats.

Under the Workplace (Health, Safety and Welfare) Regulations 1992 and considering the diversity in personal comfort levels, what is the minimum temperature guideline for maintaining a comfortable office environment?

The answer is: b) A minimum of 16°C for sedentary work

While considering employee comfort is important, the Workplace (Health, Safety and Welfare) Regulations 1992 specify minimum temperature guidelines to ensure a safe and comfortable working environment. Personal preferences can vary widely, but regulations provide a baseline standard to protect health and safety uniformly across all employees.

For sedentary work such as office work, the minimum recommended temperature is 16°C. This guideline aims to ensure that indoor workplaces are adequately heated to provide thermal comfort for employees engaged in less physically demanding tasks, and 13°C as the minimum temperature for physically demanding work.

While temperature preferences may vary seasonally, the regulations provide a baseline minimum temperature requirement regardless of the season.

Source: www.hse.gov.uk/pubns/indg244.PDF

QUESTION 58

You are asked to help set up a biological monitoring system at a yacht building company working with styrene. A biological monitoring guidance value (BMGV) is set at 1 micromol (1 μmol) urinary diamine per mol creatinine. You are asked what is likely to happen if employees have values above this level.

What is the most appropriate answer?

The answer is: d) Work practices and controls need to be investigated

A biological monitoring guidance value (BMGV) of 1 μmol urinary diamine per mol creatinine is used to evaluate exposure to isocyanates and the effectiveness of control measures. This value is not a legal limit and has no direct health implications, but serves as a benchmark for best practices. BMGVs are based on the 90th percentile value of biological monitoring data from workplaces employing good occupational hygiene practices. Where the BMGVs are exceeded, this indicates that work practices and controls need to be investigated.

Urine testing, conducted once or twice a year, helps assess exposure by measuring isocyanate breakdown products. It supplements air sampling to gauge the effectiveness of mechanical controls and should include both exposed workers and those nearby.

Option d) is the most appropriate because it directly addresses the issue of determining why values might exceed the BMGV.

BMGV are not statutory limits. They are guidance values based on best practice and not on legal requirements. Therefore, exceeding this value does not constitute a breach of legislation.

While exceeding the BMGV might indicate higher exposure to styrene, it does not imply that health effects may occur. The BMGV is a measure for assessing exposure levels and ensuring that practices remain within safe limits, but it does not necessarily correlate directly to specific health effects.

If employees' values exceed the BMGV, it suggests that the business may not be adhering to best practice standards for controlling styrene exposure. However, investigation and evaluation of the current practices are needed to come to this conclusion, making it not the most correct answer option.

Option e), that 'the employees have not been using the controls in place' is less likely because the question is not necessarily about individual adherence to controls, but rather about the overall effectiveness of the control measures in place.

Source: www.hse.gov.uk/pubns/guidance/g408.pdf

QUESTION 59

You are undertaking a workplace visit at a gardening company with students. One of your students asks you what the limit value for hand arm vibration is.

What is the most appropriate answer?

The answer is: e) 5.0 m/s² A(8)

5.0 m/s² A(8) is the legal upper limit for daily hand arm vibration exposure, according to The Control of Vibration at Work Regulations 2005. This represents the maximum amount of vibration exposure allowed for an employee per day, beyond which immediate action must be taken to reduce exposure.

0.5 m/s² A(8) is the exposure action value (EAV) for whole body vibration, not hand arm vibration. It represents a level at which employers should begin to take measures to control exposure.

1.15 m/s² A(8) is the exposure limit value (ELV) for whole body vibration. It is the maximum allowable daily exposure for whole body vibration, not for hand arm vibration.

2.5 m/s² A(8) is the exposure action value (EAV) for hand arm vibration. When exposure exceeds this level, employers must take action to reduce exposure, but it is not the legal upper limit.

4.5 m/s² A(8) is not specified in the regulations as either an action value or limit value for vibration exposure. It is not relevant to the legal requirements outlined in the Control of Vibration at Work Regulations 2005.

Source: www.hse.gov.uk/vibration/hav/advicetoemployers/responsibilities.htm

QUESTION 60

A manager notices that several employees have been coming to work despite being ill and performing below their usual standards. This decline in performance has affected overall productivity in the team.

What is the most appropriate term to describe this phenomenon?

The answer is: b) Presenteeism

Presenteeism refers to the phenomenon where employees come to work while sick and perform below their usual standards, resulting in lost productivity.

Absenteeism refers to employees not being at work due to illness or other reasons, not attending work while ill.

Job burnout refers to chronic workplace stress leading to emotional and physical exhaustion.

Work–life imbalance relates to a poor balance between work demands and personal life, not about illness-related performance at work.

Overtime refers to working beyond regular hours, which is unrelated to presenteeism.

Sources:
- www.som.org.uk/Presenteeism_during_the_COVID-19_pandemic_May_2021.pdf
- www.rospa.com/news-and-views/the-hidden-costs-of-presenteeism

QUESTION 61

A worker complains of eye discomfort and distraction while working on a computer screen for long periods in a brightly lit office. The lighting in the room causes a part of the visual field to be much brighter than the rest. Although the worker's vision is not directly impaired, they report feeling irritated and visually fatigued.

Which term best describes the glare this worker is experiencing?

The answer is: c) Discomfort glare

Glare occurs when one part of the visual field is significantly brighter than the average brightness to which the visual system is adapted, leading to symptoms such as discomfort, annoyance and visual fatigue. Unlike disability glare, which directly interferes with vision, discomfort glare does not impair vision but can cause irritability and distraction. Both types of glare can come from the same source, such as bright office lighting or reflections on screens.

Source: https://books.hse.gov.uk/gempdf/hsg38.pdf

QUESTION 62

You see a student midwife who has just started her clinical rotation. She was in the birthing suite when she noticed a burning sensation and red swellings on her hands. The rash resolved itself within 24 hours of onset.

You suspect that this was related to wearing latex gloves.

What is the most likely type of reaction in this condition?

The answer is: a) Type 1 hypersensitivity

Type 1 hypersensitivity is an immediate allergic reaction mediated by IgE antibodies. It typically involves symptoms such as burning sensation, hives (urticaria) and red swellings (wheals), which occur rapidly after exposure to the allergen and resolve within hours. Latex allergy is a common example of type 1 hypersensitivity.

Type 2 hypersensitivity involves IgG or IgM antibodies binding to antigens on the surface of cells, leading to cell destruction. Conditions such as haemolytic anaemia or Goodpasture syndrome are examples. It does not typically present with immediate skin reactions like those described in this scenario.

Type 3 hypersensitivity involves immune complex formation (antigen–antibody complexes) that deposit in various tissues, leading to inflammation and tissue damage. Examples include systemic lupus erythematosus and post-streptococcal glomerulonephritis. This type of hypersensitivity does not fit the acute skin symptoms seen in latex allergy.

Type 4 hypersensitivity is a delayed-type hypersensitivity mediated by T cells, leading to symptoms that develop hours to days after exposure. Examples include contact dermatitis and the tuberculin skin test reaction. While latex allergy can also cause type 4 hypersensitivity reactions, the immediate nature of the symptoms described here suggests a type 1 reaction.

There are only four types of hypersensitivity reaction – type 5 does not exist.

Source: Sadhra, S., Bray, A.J. and Boorman, S. (eds) (2022) *Oxford Handbook of Occupational Health*, 3rd edition

QUESTION 63

You receive a call from an occupational technician who is on site undertaking pure tone audiometry as part of routine health surveillance assessment for noise exposure. He describes an audiogram for a 45-year-old factory worker attending for his 3-year review; the summation of the hearing levels obtained at 1, 2, 3, 4 and 6 kHz indicates a new Category 3 result in both ears.

What action would it be most appropriate to take, based on this result?

The answer is: d) Further review by an OHP

New Category 3 result in pure tone audiometry indicates a hearing threshold shift requiring referral for a medical assessment by an appropriately trained doctor, such as an occupational physician. This assessment is crucial to evaluate potential occupational noise-induced hearing loss and determine appropriate follow-up actions.

The referral can happen virtually or be a 'paper' review exercise rather than requiring face-to-face examination. The essential requirement is for the doctor to have all relevant information available to them to make a judgement alongside appropriate competence to make a judgement.

An ear, nose and throat (ENT) specialist may be involved in further assessment. The initial referral for a Category 3 result is typically to an appropriately trained occupational health physician for occupational health surveillance purposes.

Further review of the workplace and review of the controls may be a further step if noise-induced hearing loss is diagnosed.

Sources:
- www.som.org.uk/sites/som.org.uk/files/SOM_UKHCA_Position_Statement_Noise_Health_Surveillance_Guidance_May_23.pdf
- www.hse.gov.uk/pubns/priced/l108.pdf
- www.som.org.uk/sites/som.org.uk/files/Supplementary_Guidance_on_Interpreting_an_Audiogram_for_Indications_of_Occupational_NIHL_Sept_2024.pdf

QUESTION 64

Oskar applies for a job as a scaffolder. On the application form, he is asked whether there is any reason why he cannot climb ladders or work at a height, both tasks intrinsic to the job. Oskar discloses that he has epilepsy, which he manages with medication. The employer is concerned about the safety implications of Oskar working at heights and decides to conduct a risk assessment to determine if the work is hazardous for him.

As an occupational health physician advising the employer, what is the best course of action to ensure compliance with the Equality Act 2010 while addressing the safety concerns?

The answer is: c) Conduct a thorough risk assessment to determine if there are reasonable adjustments that could enable Oskar to safely perform the job

Employers are allowed to ask questions about health prior to the job offer, if it is necessary to establish whether the applicant can carry out a function that is intrinsic to the work concerned, as long as they are compliant with the Equality Act 2010.

While the Equality Act requires reasonable adjustments, these must be feasible and practical. A risk assessment must be conducted first to determine what adjustments are reasonable and whether the role can be safely performed by the individual.

If the ability to work at heights is intrinsic to the role, excluding Oskar from such tasks would likely make it impossible for him to fulfil the job requirements. A risk assessment is necessary to explore feasible adjustments first.

Rejecting the application outright without a thorough risk assessment and consideration of reasonable adjustments would be discriminatory and non-compliant with the Equality Act 2010.

Source: https://assets.publishing.service.gov.uk/media/5a79b5d440f0b642860da26f/employment-health-questions.pdf

QUESTION 65

You conduct a walkthrough survey at a mechanics shop and ask to see the risk assessment, but the employer does not have one documented.

How many employees does an employer need to have before there is a legal requirement to document a risk assessment?

The answer is: c) 5

Employers are legally required to document their risk assessments if they have five or more employees. This includes identifying hazards, determining who might be harmed, and outlining how the risks are being controlled. For businesses with fewer than five employees, risk assessments must still be conducted, but they do not need to be documented.

Source: www.hse.gov.uk/simple-health-safety/risk/steps-needed-to-manage-risk.htm#_Record_your_findings

QUESTION 66

A company is developing a strategy to manage and reduce employee absenteeism.

Which of the following statements best reflects the importance of past sickness absence?

The answer is: b) Past sickness absence is a key indicator of future absence risk, with a higher number of past absences suggesting an increased risk of future absences

Research and evidence show that past sickness absence is a strong predictor of future absence risk.

Source: Hobson, J. and Smedley, J. (eds) (2019) *Fitness for Work: the medical aspects*, 6th edition. Oxford University Press

QUESTION 67

A warehouse packer who suffers from Raynaud's disease complains that the warehouse is too cold.

What is the minimum temperature requirement for this workplace?

The answer is: b) 13°C

Under the Workplace (Health, Safety and Welfare) Regulations there is a legal obligation on employers to provide a 'reasonable' temperature in the workplace.

It suggests that the minimum temperature in a workplace should normally be at least 16°C. If the work involves vigorous physical effort, such as a warehouse, the temperature should be at least 13°C.

QUESTION 68

You are an occupational health advisor for a manufacturing company where employees are frequently exposed to metal fumes from welding. The company is considering offering pneumococcal vaccinations to all employees to reduce the risk of pneumococcal diseases. Some employees have expressed concerns about the vaccine and are unsure if they want to receive it.

What is the most appropriate advice to provide the company regarding the pneumococcal vaccination policy for employees exposed to metal fumes?

The answer is: e) The pneumococcal vaccine should be presented as optional for employees, with assurance that they will not face any negative consequences if they choose not to receive it

The vaccine should be offered as an optional measure, and employees must not feel coerced or discriminated against based on their decision to accept or decline the vaccination. It is essential to respect the autonomy of employees and ensure they have the freedom to make informed choices about their health without fear of repercussions or discrimination in the workplace. Strongly encouraging employees to take the vaccine may be seen as coercion.

Source: www.hse.gov.uk/pubns/eis44.pdf

QUESTION 69

You see a student nurse in your screening clinic who is due to start work on the paediatric ward. As part of routine screening, you note that her interferon gamma release assay (IGRA) test is negative but she has not been vaccinated against tuberculosis (TB).

Which one of the following is the most appropriate next step prior to BCG vaccination?

The answer is: a) HIV test

If an employee new to the NHS has no (or inconclusive) evidence of prior BCG vaccination, a Mantoux tuberculin skin test or interferon gamma test should be performed.

Employees who will be working with patients or clinical specimens and who are Mantoux tuberculin skin test or interferon gamma test negative should have an individual risk assessment for HIV infection before BCG vaccination is given.

BCG vaccine is absolutely contraindicated in all HIV-positive persons regardless of CD4 cell count, antiretroviral therapy (ART) use, viral load and clinical status.

No further investigation is warranted if they have no evidence of TB.

Source: https://assets.publishing.service.gov.uk/media/5a7ed8d5e5274a2e87db2479/health_clearance_tuberculosis_hepatitis_hiv.pdf

QUESTION 70

A healthcare worker sustains a needlestick injury while treating a patient known to be positive for hepatitis B.

What is the estimated risk of hepatitis B transmission from the patient to the healthcare worker?

The answer is: b) Up to 30%

The risk of hepatitis B transmission from a needlestick injury is significantly higher compared to other blood-borne viruses, with an estimated risk of up to 30%. This elevated risk underscores the importance of immediate post-exposure prophylaxis, which includes the hepatitis B vaccine and potentially hepatitis B immunoglobulin (HBIg), depending on the healthcare worker's immunisation status.

Source: www.hse.gov.uk/biosafety/blood-borne-viruses/how-deal-exposure-incident.htm

QUESTION 71

You are helping a student with a research problem. They have some queries about confidence intervals.

If a study quotes a 95% confidence interval, which one of the following statements is true?

The answer is: b) There is a 5% chance of the true value lying outside these limits

The 95% confidence interval (CI) indicates that the true value has a 95% chance of lying within this range. It is represented on a forest plot as a horizontal line.

Source: Sadhra, S., Bray, A.J. and Boorman, S. (eds) (2022) *Oxford Handbook of Occupational Health*, 3rd edition

QUESTION 72

You are an occupational health physician for a corporate office. You see Ms Floyd, a data analyst who works long hours at a computer. She complains of frequent eye strain, headaches and neck discomfort. Ms Floyd mentions that due to her workload, she often skips breaks and continues working at her desk for extended periods without interruption.

Based on Ms Floyd's symptoms and the regulations concerning display screen equipment (DSE) users, what is the most appropriate advice you should provide regarding breaks?

The answer is: c) Short breaks taken frequently are more beneficial than longer breaks less often

The Health and Safety (Display Screen Equipment) Regulations 1992, as amended by the Health and Safety (Miscellaneous Amendments) Regulations 2002, say employers must plan work so there are breaks or changes of activity for employees who are DSE users. There is no legal guidance about how long and how often breaks should be for DSE work. Taking shorter breaks more frequently is more beneficial than longer breaks taken less frequently. Ideally, users should be able to choose when to take breaks. In most jobs it is possible to stop DSE work to do other tasks, such as going to meetings or making phone calls. If there are no natural changes of activity in a job, employers should plan rest breaks. Breaks or changes of activity should allow users to get up from their workstations and move around, or at least stretch and change posture. Break-monitoring software can remind users to take regular breaks, but employers are still responsible for making sure work activities are properly planned and that users take suitable breaks.

Sources:
- www.hse.gov.uk/pubns/books/l26.htm
- Sadhra, S., Bray, A.J. and Boorman, S. (eds) (2022) *Oxford Handbook of Occupational Health*, 3rd edition

QUESTION 73

You are an occupational health physician who has been asked to provide evidence for an employment tribunal regarding a case where a worker alleges unfair dismissal due to a disability. Your role involves providing expert opinions on the worker's health and its impact on their employment.

What is the primary function of the employment tribunal in this context?

The answer is: c) To make legally binding decisions on disputes related to employment rights

The employment tribunal's primary function is to resolve disputes related to employment rights. This includes making legally binding decisions on cases involving unfair dismissal, discrimination and other employment-related issues. It assesses the evidence provided, including expert opinions, to determine if the employer's actions were lawful and if any statutory obligations were met.

Mediation services, counselling and workplace inspections are outside the scope of the employment tribunal's responsibilities.

Answers to Mock exam 2

QUESTION 74

A 50-year-old radiation safety officer is conducting a training session for new staff at a hospital that uses various types of radiological equipment. The officer needs to explain the different penetrating potentials of radiation types, to ensure that appropriate safety measures and shielding are in place. The staff ask for clarification on which type of radiation requires the most substantial shielding due to its high penetrating power.

Which of the following types of radiation has the greatest penetrating ability and therefore requires the most substantial shielding?

The answer is: c) Gamma rays

The penetrating ability of ionising radiation is an important consideration in the type of shielding needed.

Gamma rays have the highest penetrating ability among the types of radiation listed. They can easily pass through the human body and require dense shielding materials, such as lead or thick concrete, to block their effects.

Alpha particles have low penetration power and can be stopped by a sheet of paper or the outer layer of the skin.

Beta particles have moderate penetration and can be shielded by materials such as plastic or aluminium.

X-rays, though similar to gamma rays, generally have lower energy and require less dense shielding compared to gamma rays.

Positrons, the antimatter counterparts of electrons, have a similar penetrating ability to beta particles. They interact with electrons in the surrounding matter, leading to annihilation and the emission of gamma rays, but the positrons themselves are not as penetrating as gamma rays.

Source: https://oshwiki.osha.europa.eu/en/themes/ionising-radiation-workplaces

QUESTION 75

You see a 50-year-old farmer with a 3-month history of cough and shortness of breath that he feels is worse at work. His symptoms improved during a recent

3-week holiday. He also reports malaise and weight loss. He does not smoke and has an otherwise unremarkable medical history.

What is the most likely diagnosis?

The answer is: b) Hypersensitivity pneumonitis (HP)

Based on the presented case, hypersensitivity pneumonitis (HP), also known as extrinsic allergic alveolitis (EAA), is the most likely diagnosis due to the correlation of symptoms with workplace exposures of a farmer and the systemic symptoms described.

Occupational asthma and obliterative bronchiolitis are important considerations but are less likely given the specific context and symptomatology. COPD and lung cancer are less probable given the patient's non-smoking status and symptom improvement during a holiday.

Further diagnostic testing should be pursued to confirm the diagnosis.

The following are important differential diagnoses:

Occupational asthma (OA):
- Symptoms: cough, wheezing and breathlessness worsened by workplace exposure and improved away from work.
- Differential: needs to be considered, but lacks the systemic symptoms (malaise, weight loss) and improvement after holiday suggests a more chronic and systemic response consistent with HP.

Chronic obstructive pulmonary disease (COPD):
- Symptoms: chronic cough, sputum production and breathlessness.
- Exposure: occupational exposures of a farmer (including grain and organic dusts) can cause COPD, but the absence of a smoking history and rapid symptom improvement during holidays makes COPD less likely.

Lung cancer:
- Symptoms: chronic cough, weight loss and malaise are concerning, but the improvement of symptoms away from work makes cancer less likely.

Obliterative bronchiolitis:
- Symptoms: insidious onset of cough and breathlessness, often with rapid and fixed airflow obstruction.

Source: Sadhra, S., Bray, A.J. and Boorman, S. (eds) (2022) *Oxford Handbook of Occupational Health*, 3rd edition

QUESTION 76

You are an occupational health professional starting a new role at a large healthcare organisation. As part of your induction, you are informed about the safeguarding training requirements necessary for your role. The organisation highlights the importance of ensuring that all staff working in occupational health are appropriately trained to identify and act on safeguarding concerns involving children and vulnerable individuals.

What is the minimum level of safeguarding training required for occupational health professionals?

The answer is: b) Level 2 safeguarding training

Safeguarding is "Protecting health, wellbeing and human rights; enabling [people] to live free from harm, abuse and neglect. It is an integral part of providing high-quality health care. Safeguarding children, young people and adults is a collective responsibility." (NHS England)

OH practitioners may become involved in safeguarding of children or vulnerable adults when:
1. There is a concern that an employee may be putting someone at harm – there may be a statement of intent of neglect or harm or disclosure of abuse/neglect
2. Condition or circumstances may put someone at risk outside of the workplace, e.g. severe mental illness
3. Employee may be a risk to children in the workplace.

Occupational health professionals are required to complete Level 2 safeguarding training to ensure they can identify and respond appropriately to concerns about the welfare of children and vulnerable individuals. This competency aligns with intercollegiate guidance and emphasises the importance of recognising potential safeguarding issues in the workplace and taking appropriate action.

Source: https://childprotection.rcpch.ac.uk/resources/safeguarding-children-guidelines-for-occupational-health-professionals

QUESTION 77

You have been asked to review a spirometry test performed by a student technician for asbestos health surveillance, and the results are shown in the graph below.

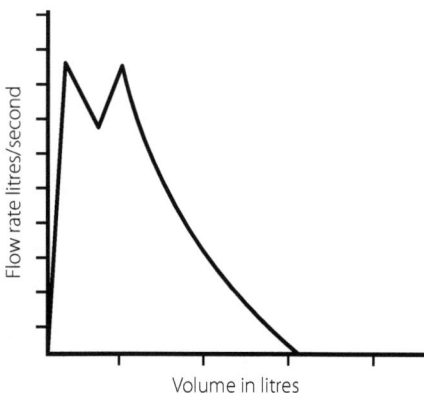

What is the most likely cause of the spirometry pattern observed in this graph?

The answer is: b) Extra breath taken during the test

An extra breath taken during the test is suboptimal and therefore the test needs to performed again.

Source: www.brit-thoracic.org.uk/media/70454/spirometry_e-guide_2013.pdf

QUESTION 78

You see a 42-year-old construction worker who has worked with pneumatic drills for 1 year. He is complaining of numbness and tingling in the little and ring finger of his dominant hand, which he feels is associated with using the drill. He does notice that it also occurs when he is lifting weights at the gym. He is a smoker of 10 cigarettes a day since he was 20 years old.

From the information above, what is the most likely diagnosis?

The answer is: b) Cubital tunnel syndrome

A thorough clinical history, physical examination and appropriate diagnostic tests are crucial to distinguish HAVS from these conditions. Each has unique characteristics and patterns that can help in accurate diagnosis and management.

Cubital tunnel syndrome (ulnar nerve syndrome): this involves compression of the ulnar nerve at the elbow, leading to symptoms such as numbness and tingling in the ring and little fingers. Unlike HAVS, cubital tunnel syndrome symptoms are often exacerbated by elbow flexion.

The differential diagnosis of hand arm vibration syndrome (HAVS) includes:

Carpal tunnel syndrome (CTS): caused by compression of the median nerve at the wrist.

Raynaud's disease: involves episodic digital ischaemia in response to cold or stress, leading to colour changes (white, blue, red) in fingers.

Thoracic outlet syndrome (TOS): results from compression of nerves or blood vessels between the collarbone and first rib, causing arm pain, numbness and weakness.

Peripheral neuropathy: caused by systemic conditions such as diabetes, it leads to numbness, tingling and pain in a 'glove and stocking' distribution.

Source: www.som.org.uk/sites/som.org.uk/files/HAVS_Guidance_updated_March_2023.pdf

QUESTION 79

You are an NHS occupational health physician. You are evaluating a hospital porter and need more information to guide your decision-making regarding his fitness for work. You notice that he is currently under the care of several specialists at the hospital where you work.

What is the best way to obtain the information that you need?

The answer is: d) Obtain the hospital porter's consent to request information from his specialists

According to GMC guidelines, you must not abuse your privileged position as a doctor to gain access to a patient's hospital or medical records without proper authorisation. Clinical information should be requested with the patient's consent through the appropriate channels. The most appropriate action is to obtain explicit consent from the hospital porter to request information from his specialists. This respects patient confidentiality and follows the ethical and legal requirements for handling personal medical information.

Source: www.fom.ac.uk/wp-content/uploads/GOMP_2017_Web.pdf

QUESTION 80

You are writing hospital guidance for the management of healthcare workers who accidentally sustain needlestick injuries.

What is the most appropriate immediate action following the injury?

The answer is: c) Gently encourage the wound to bleed and wash it with soap and water

The correct immediate response following a needlestick injury is to gently encourage the wound to bleed and wash it with soap and water. Scrubbing or sucking the wound should be avoided, as it may damage tissue or increase the risk of infection. It is not necessary to keep the needle for testing, as blood-borne virus testing is typically conducted on the source patient. The needle should be safely disposed in a sharps container and never re-sheathed to prevent further injury.

Source: www.hse.gov.uk/biosafety/blood-borne-viruses/how-deal-exposure-incident.htm

QUESTIONS for Mock exam 3

QUESTION 1

You are leading an orientation session for new occupational health (OH) practitioners in a large industrial company. During the session, one of the practitioners asks about the legal framework that governs workplace safety and health.

Which of the following best describes the difference between an Act and a Regulation?

a) An Act provides specific, detailed rules for occupational health, while a Regulation is a broad statement of principles
b) An Act establishes the overall legal framework, while a Regulation is a detailed rule made under the Act to implement and enforce its provisions
c) An Act is legally binding, while a Regulation is a set of optional guidelines that employers may choose to follow
d) There is no difference between an Act and a Regulation
e) An Act is a temporary measure, while a Regulation is permanent and unchangeable

QUESTION 2

You are advising an employer who is facing a conflict between medical opinions regarding an employee's fitness for work. The employee's GP has stated on the 'fit' note that the individual is unfit for work, while the OH professional has provided a robust report after gaining information from the employee's specialist indicating the employee is fit to return with reasonable adjustments. The employer is unsure which medical opinion to prioritise in making their decision.

What is the most reasonable action for the employer to take in this situation?

a) Rely on the employee's GP's opinion, as it reflects the individual's personal medical history and tribunals typically consider this a reasonable approach
b) Seek legal advice before making any decisions, as conflicting opinions may lead to litigation, which should be avoided at all cost
c) Follow the recommendation of the OH professional, as tribunals typically consider this a reasonable approach
d) Request a joint consultation between the employee's GP and the OH professional and the employee to reach a consensus, as tribunals typically consider this a reasonable approach
e) Seek a third opinion from another OH professional

QUESTION 3

An occupational health physician (OHP) is evaluating an employee with a medical condition. The employer seeks clarification on whether the employee's condition meets the legal definition of disability under the Equality Act (EqA).

Which entity has the authority to make a final legal determination regarding whether an employee's condition satisfies the definition of disability under the EqA?

a) The occupational health (OH) professional
b) The Human Resources (HR) department of the employer
c) The employment tribunal (ET)
d) The employee's primary care physician
e) The employee's specialist physician

QUESTION 4

You are evaluating a 20-year-old warehouse operative who has just had his driver's licence revoked following a recent seizure. Prior to the recent seizure, he had been seizure-free for the past 10 years. Management is seeking advice on whether he is fit to undertake his role, which involves manual handling and forklift truck driving.

Which of the following options is the most appropriate advice regarding the fitness of the warehouse operative to undertake his role following the seizure?

a) Fit to undertake full role
b) Restrict from manual handling
c) Fit to undertake forklift truck driving under supervision
d) Fit to undertake manual handling with manual handling aids
e) Restrict from forklift truck driving

QUESTION 5

You are consulting with a 55-year-old gardener who is seeking advice on returning to work after a total hip replacement. He is extremely worried that he will not be able to return to his job following the operation.

What percentage of individuals manage to return to their original work after a total hip replacement?

a) 50–70% of patients manage to return to their original work
b) 10–20% of patients manage to return to their original work
c) 80–100% of patients manage to return to their original work
d) 100% of patients manage to return to their original work
e) Less than 50% of patients manage to return to their original work

QUESTION 6

You are reviewing the case of a healthcare worker (HCW) living with hepatitis B virus (HBV) who has been cleared to perform exposure-prone procedures (EPPs).

Who is primarily responsible for the ongoing monitoring of this HCW to ensure compliance with health and safety regulations?

a) The healthcare worker's line manager
b) The treating physician of the healthcare worker
c) The hospital infection control team
d) The accredited specialist in occupational medicine
e) The Human Resources department

QUESTION 7

During a teaching session for medical students, you are asked a question about the role of an occupational hygienist. The students want to understand the primary responsibilities of an occupational hygienist within the workplace.

Which of the following best describes the primary role of an occupational hygienist?

a) To design or modify the work to fit the worker
b) To apply psychology to the workplace to improve the effectiveness of organisations and the job satisfaction of employees
c) To administer medical treatment for respiratory conditions caused by workplace exposures
d) To undertake health surveillance procedures
e) To identify, evaluate and manage work-related hazards that may contribute to employee health issues

QUESTION 8

You are an OHP who has completed an assessment of a 40-year-old construction worker with chronic knee pain. The worker requested to see a copy of the report before it was sent to their employer. You provided the report to the worker and allowed a reasonable timeframe for them to review and provide feedback. Despite this, you have not received any response from the worker within the specified period.

What is the most appropriate next step in this situation?

a) Withdraw the report as consent has not been reaffirmed

b) Wait an additional few weeks before taking any action to ensure the worker has sufficient time to respond
c) Contact the worker to follow up on their review of the report and remind them of the deadline for providing any feedback
d) Assume the worker has no concerns and send the report to the employer without further action
e) Re-send the report to the worker to ensure they have received it and then submit it to the employer once confirmed

QUESTION 9

A sanitation worker presents for an occupational health assessment. He frequently works with raw, untreated sewage and asks about vaccination recommendations to protect his health.

Which of the following is the most appropriate preventive measure for workers exposed to raw sewage?

a) Immunisation against hepatitis B
b) Immunisation against varicella zoster virus
c) Immunisation against hepatitis A
d) Immunisation against *Pneumococcus*
e) Immunisation against SARS-CoV-2

QUESTION 10

You are part of a committee which has proposed a study to look at whether exposure to nanoparticles is linked to renal failure.

The proposed study methodology data is to be obtained from groups who have been exposed, or not exposed, to nanoparticles.

Which type of study does this best describe?

a) Randomised controlled trial (RCT)
b) Case–control study
c) Cross-sectional study
d) Cohort study
e) Crossover design

QUESTION 11

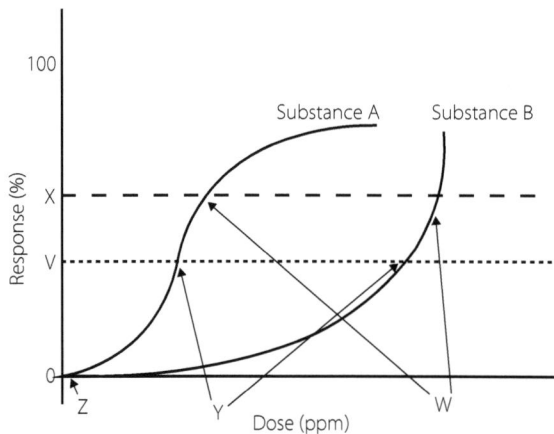

Note: ppm = parts per million

Looking at the dose–response curves, which one of the following is correct?

a) B is more potent than A
b) Y is the lowest observed level
c) V is the LD50
d) Z is the threshold level
e) W is the no observable effect level

QUESTION 12

You are the occupational physician in a large company that makes furniture. There is poor compliance with controls and you are concerned about the employees' exposure to wood dust.

Which of the following is most associated with wood dust exposure?

a) Lung cancer
b) Squamous cell carcinoma of the skin
c) Sinonasal carcinoma
d) Laryngeal cancer
e) Ovarian cancer

QUESTION 13

A 50-year-old female textile worker presents to the clinic with complaints of chest tightness, coughing, wheezing and shortness of breath that began a few months ago. She reports that these symptoms are most severe at the beginning of the work week and gradually improve by the end of the week. She notices significant relief from her symptoms during weekends and vacations when she is away from work. The patient has worked in a textile factory for the past 20 years. She has a history of smoking 10 cigarettes a day since the age of 20 but has no other known medical problems. Spirometry shows a reduced FEV_1.

What is the most likely diagnosis?

a) Occupational asthma
b) Byssinosis
c) Chronic obstructive pulmonary disease (COPD)
d) Hypersensitivity pneumonitis
e) Tuberculosis

QUESTION 14

A surgeon has been diagnosed with dry age-related macular degeneration which has become significantly worse over the last 5 months.

For this reason, their employer reviews the situation and decides they need to stop the surgeon performing operations.

The surgeon feels they are being discriminated against.

Which of the following is the best term for this?

a) Direct discrimination
b) Harassment
c) Objective justification
d) Positive action
e) Victimisation

QUESTION 15

You are conducting a remote consultation with a 54-year-old man who recently experienced an uncomplicated cerebrovascular event while abroad on business. The man wishes to return home to his family, and his employer is seeking guidance on when he can safely travel by air.

What is the most appropriate advice regarding air travel following an uncomplicated cerebrovascular event?

a) Air travel is contraindicated for at least 3 days after an uncomplicated cerebrovascular event
b) Air travel is contraindicated for 7–10 days after an uncomplicated cerebrovascular event
c) Air travel is safe immediately after an uncomplicated cerebrovascular event, provided the patient feels well
d) Air travel is contraindicated for 14–21 days after an uncomplicated cerebrovascular event
e) Air travel is contraindicated until a full cardiac evaluation is completed, regardless of the time elapsed

QUESTION 16

You are evaluating a 36-year-old construction worker who has been escalated to Tier 4 vibration health surveillance. He presents with sensory disturbances in the little and ring fingers, clawing of the hand, and atrophy of the hypothenar eminence. The fixed flexion test is positive.

What is the most likely diagnosis?

a) Carpal tunnel syndrome
b) Cubital tunnel syndrome
c) Guyon tunnel syndrome
d) HAVS (hand arm vibration syndrome)
e) Pronator teres syndrome

QUESTION 17

An individual who is self-employed has sustained a work-related injury and is considering applying for Industrial Injuries Disablement Benefit (IIDB) and asks you about it.

Based on the eligibility criteria, which one of the following statements is correct?

a) The individual can apply for IIDB if they provide evidence that their injury is directly related to any employment
b) The individual cannot apply for IIDB because self-employed individuals are not eligible for this benefit
c) The individual can apply for IIDB as long as they were not an apprentice at the time of diagnosis
d) The individual cannot apply for IIDB if they are no longer working
e) The individual cannot apply for IIDB if they are no longer working in an industry related to the disease

QUESTION 18

You undertake a workplace visit at a material recovery facility. It appears to be noisy, but no hygiene measurements are available. The noise appears intrusive, but normal conversation is possible. The supervisor informs you that the noise level is like this for the full 6-hour shift.

What would you estimate the noise level to be in your report?

a) 80 dB(A)
b) 85 dB(A)
c) 90 dB(A)
d) Over 90 dB(A)
e) Under 80 dB(A)

QUESTION 19

You are delivering a lecture on screening tests and their effectiveness in OH settings. A trainee asks about the factors that influence the positive predictive value (PPV) of a test.

Which one of the following statements about the PPV of a screening test is correct?

a) PPV decreases as disease prevalence increases
b) PPV increases with increasing sensitivity of the screening test
c) PPV decreases with increasing sensitivity of the screening test
d) PPV remains the same regardless of the sensitivity of the screening test
e) PPV remains constant regardless of disease prevalence

QUESTION 20

You are an OHP conducting a telephone consultation with Mr Patel, a 40-year-old employee seeking advice on managing stress-related symptoms at work. Mr Patel has signed the consent form sent with the referral to take part in the consultation.

What is the best practice for taking consent in remote occupational health consultations?

a) Proceed with the consultation assuming implicit consent, unless Mr Patel explicitly objects during the consultation
b) Request Mr Patel to send an email confirming his consent after the consultation
c) The employee will have been sent a consent form prior to your consultation which has been signed – this is sufficient to proceed
d) Send the report to the employee for prior viewing and confirm consent at this point
e) Record Mr Patel's verbal consent in the consultation notes contemporaneously

QUESTION 21

Dr Grimes, an OH consultant, has been asked to review the devised plan for a new out-of-hours service at a large hospital. The goal is to ensure that the new shift patterns are safe and effective for both staff and patients. The current plan includes forward rotating shifts, timing shifts to avoid starting before 7am, limiting shift duration to 12 hours, providing adequate rest breaks, and ensuring compliance with the Working Time Regulations 1998.

Based on the principles of effective shift design, what is the most appropriate recommendation for Dr Grimes to make?

a) Allow staff to sleep on site after their shift if they work more than an 11-hour shift, to ensure they receive adequate rest
b) Consider lighting and temperature adjustments during night shifts
c) Mandate that staff do not work beyond their shift length, so that they do not exceed the Working Time Regulations 1998
d) Ban shift swapping, to ensure staff get necessary rest periods and do not work excessive hours
e) Provide vending machines so that staff have access to affordable food in their breaks

QUESTION 22

You are providing a training session for managers on employer responsibilities and their duty of care to their employees. During the session, you explain the 'eggshell skull' principle.

Which one of the following does the 'eggshell skull' principle imply for employers?

a) Employers must treat all employees equally regardless of their health conditions
b) Employees with pre-existing conditions must take full responsibility for their own safety
c) Employers owe a higher duty of care to employees with known vulnerabilities
d) Pre-placement health checks are optional and not necessary
e) Employers are exempt from liability if an employee does not disclose their condition

QUESTION 23

An occupational hygienist is measuring sound levels in a workplace to assess potential hearing risks. The professional explains that the human ear is more sensitive to certain frequencies than others, and sound measurements should consider this sensitivity to obtain accurate readings.

When measuring sound levels in the workplace to evaluate potential hearing risks, which weighting should be used?

a) B-weighting
b) C-weighting
c) D-weighting
d) A-weighting
e) Linear weighting

QUESTION 24

You are asked to advise a group of engineers who work with rosin flux based on a review of a recently performed risk assessment.

Occupational hygiene measurements show that the time-weighted average (TWA) (8h) is 0.04 mg/m^3

Workplace exposure limit (WEL): 8h TWA rosin = 0.05 mg/m^3

Which one of the following is the most appropriate next step, based on the hygiene result, to mitigate the risk?

a) Conduct periodic monitoring and review of control measures
b) Exposure should be reduced to the lowest level reasonably practicable
c) Implement health surveillance for workers exposed to rosin flux
d) Provide additional training and information to workers
e) No further action is needed as the exposure is controlled to below the WEL

QUESTION 25

Mr Hassan was referred for fitness to attend a disciplinary. He had no underlying medical concerns. You discussed the importance of meeting with the employer to resolve the issue as soon as possible, as delay could actually cause more harm. Mr Hassan agreed to this and consented to the report being sent to HR. He also said he wanted to see the report before it was sent, and gave you an email address to use. You advised that when he received the report, he would have 48 hours in which to respond. Mr Hassan did not respond to OH or make any comment on the report within the 48-hour time period.

What is the most appropriate next step?

a) Send the report to HR on the basis of the consent given during the consultation
b) Withhold the report, as consent is needed to release this to HR
c) Contact the employee via an alternative method, in case his email address is incorrect
d) Ask the employer to contact the employee
e) Resend the report to his email address as a reminder

QUESTION 26

You are conducting a workshop on disability discrimination for a group of Human Resources professionals. During the session, a question arises about whether an individual who has recovered from a health condition can still be considered disabled under the Equality Act 2010.

Which one of the following statements is true regarding the classification of a person as disabled under the Equality Act 2010?

a) A person can only be classified as disabled if they are currently suffering from an illness or condition
b) A person who has recovered can still be classified as disabled if all criteria for disability are met and the condition existed after the Equality Act 2010 came into effect
c) Disability classification is only based on current health conditions and does not consider past illnesses or conditions
d) If a person recovers from a disability, they are no longer protected under the Equality Act 2010
e) A person can be retrospectively classified as disabled regardless of when the condition occurred

QUESTION 27

You are assessing a worker with a history of prolonged use of vibrating hand tools and symptoms suggestive of hand arm vibration syndrome (HAVS).

What grading system is commonly used to evaluate the severity of vascular and sensorineural deficits in HAVS?

a) Epworth score
b) International consensus score

c) Stockholm Workshop Scale
d) Glasgow Coma Scale
e) DASH score

QUESTION 28

You are reviewing the viral load results of an obstetrician who is HIV positive under your care. The viral load is reported as 2000 copies/ml.

What is the most appropriate next action?

a) Review next set of blood tests in 3 months
b) Restrict the obstetrician from performing EPPs with immediate effect
c) Restrict the obstetrician from performing all clinical duties
d) Recommend a repeat viral load to confirm the result
e) Allow the obstetrician to continue working with additional personal protective equipment

QUESTION 29

You speak to a manager who wants to refer an individual who is neurodifferent for advice on adjustments.

What is the most common functional impairment in neurodifferent individuals?

a) Managing stress
b) Managing intense emotions
c) Memory/concentration
d) Organisation and time management
e) Written communication speed

QUESTION 30

You see a 65-year-old electrician referred with work-related stress. He tells you that he thinks his employer wants him to retire.

Which one of the following statements is accurate regarding retirement age?

a) Employers are required to retire employees at age 65
b) There is a mandatory retirement age of 65 in most workplaces

c) There is a voluntary retirement age of 65 in most workplaces
d) There is no mandatory age of retirement
e) Employees must retire by age 70 if they work in a safety-critical role

QUESTION 31

You are teaching a group of students about the principles of radiological protection. A student wants clarification about the effect of distance on radiation intensity.

What is the effect if you double the distance from the source of radiation?

a) The radiation intensity remains the same
b) The radiation intensity doubles
c) The radiation intensity is reduced to one-fourth
d) The radiation intensity is reduced to one-half
e) The radiation intensity increases fourfold

QUESTION 32

A 45-year-old factory worker is undergoing routine health screening as part of an OH assessment. The company uses two different tests to screen for a common industrial disease. One test is known for its high sensitivity, the other test is noted for its high specificity.

Which of the following best describes the role of sensitivity and specificity in occupational health screening?

a) Sensitivity is the ability to correctly identify workers who do not have the disease, while specificity is the ability to correctly identify workers who have the disease
b) Sensitivity is the ability to correctly identify workers who have the disease, while specificity is the ability to correctly identify workers who do not have the disease
c) Sensitivity and specificity both refer to the ability to identify workers with the disease, but in different ways
d) Sensitivity and specificity are interchangeable and do not impact the effectiveness of health screenings
e) Sensitivity measures the rate of false negatives, while specificity measures the rate of false positives

QUESTION 33

A factory worker who recently moved to your area presents to your clinic with a history of stannosis. This condition was diagnosed in his previous job where he was exposed to dust.

Which one of the following causes stannosis?

a) Tin dust
b) Silica dust
c) Asbestos fibres
d) Coal dust
e) Beryllium dust

QUESTION 34

You are undertaking a complex ill-health retirement case in which a 55-year-old employee has been absent from work for one year with fibromyalgia. The clinician is considering supporting ill-health retirement but wants to ensure the decision is based on the highest quality evidence available.

Which of the following represents the highest level of evidence to guide your decision?

a) Expert opinion
b) Case–control studies
c) Randomised controlled trials (RCTs)
d) Systematic reviews
e) Cohort studies

QUESTION 35

You are advising an employer about the increased vulnerabilities of young workers.

Which of the following would be considered a young worker?

a) An individual aged under 21
b) An individual aged 18
c) An individual aged under 18

d) An individual aged under 16
e) An individual aged 21 but still in training

QUESTION 36

You are assisting an employer in setting up a drug and alcohol screening process for employees in safety-critical roles. A manager asks about the importance of a "chain of custody" in this context.

Which of the following best describes "chain of custody"?

a) The process for managing the recall of employees for testing
b) A document verifying employee consent for testing
c) The process for managing the collection, handling, storage and testing of samples
d) The process for disciplining employees who test positive
e) A process for managing test results within the Human Resources department to ensure confidentiality

QUESTION 37

A 52-year-old bus driver is diagnosed with a medical condition that may impact his ability to drive safely.

Which one of the following has the duty to inform the Driver and Vehicle Licensing Agency (DVLA)?

a) Employer
b) Occupational health physician (OHP)
c) GP
d) Specialist clinician
e) Licence holder

QUESTION 38

A 25-year-old chef has experienced three episodes of diarrhoea and has informed his manager, who then seeks your advice in advance to manage the chef's return to work.

What is the most appropriate response to give?

a) He can return in 36 hours after his symptoms start
b) He can continue to work with increased hand hygiene measures
c) He can return to work 48 hours after his symptoms stop
d) He needs medical clearance to return
e) He can return to work 36 hours after his symptoms stop

QUESTION 39

A receptionist in the emergency department was bitten by a patient known to be infected with hepatitis B. She is anxious about the risk of transmission and asks about the effectiveness of the hepatitis B vaccination course she started within the appropriate timeframe.

What is the effectiveness of the hepatitis B vaccination in preventing hepatitis B infection when given as post-exposure prophylaxis?

a) Less than 50%
b) 60–70%
c) 75–85%
d) >95%
e) 90%

QUESTION 40

A 55-year-old worker presents to the OH clinic for health surveillance. Spirometry is performed and the flow-volume loop shown below is observed.

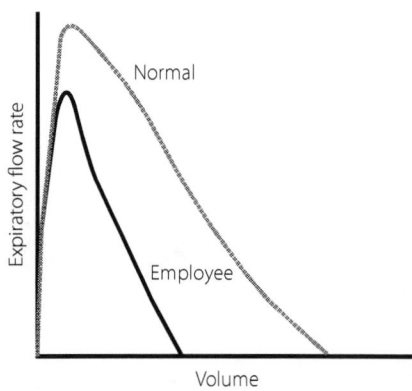

Which occupational hazard is most likely to cause the pulmonary function result shown?

a) Silica
b) Flour dust
c) Arsine
d) Benzene
e) Rosin

QUESTION 41

You are reviewing the occupational health risks associated with air conditioning engineers.

Which one of the following pathogens are air conditioning engineers more likely to be exposed to than the general population, due to their occupation?

a) *Plasmodium vivax*
b) *Mycobacterium tuberculosis*
c) *Streptococcus pneumoniae*
d) *Legionella pneumophila*
e) *Borrelia burgdorferi*

QUESTION 42

You are part of a working group discussing the potential classification of osteoarthritis as a prescribed disease in a platinum extraction process due to exposure to substance 'X' at the Industrial Injuries Advisory Council (IIAC).

The evidence does not appear clear-cut and the group is looking at any evidence of an increased relative risk of the disease in the occupational group.

What evidence of increased relative risk is needed to support the designation of a prescribed disease?

a) More than 1
b) More than 2
c) More than 3
d) More than 4
e) More than 5

QUESTION 43

You have started as the OP at a toothpaste factory and your first task is to help the business determine their first aid requirements. The factory employs 200 people.

What is the minimum number of first aiders needed in this factory?

a) 1
b) 4
c) 8
d) 12
e) 20

QUESTION 44

A company is reviewing its policies on managing employee sickness absence. It is referring to guidelines from the National Institute for Health and Care Excellence (NICE) to determine what constitutes long-term sickness absence.

According to NICE, how is long-term sickness absence defined?

a) Absences from work lasting 3 or more months
b) Absences from work lasting 1 year or more
c) Absences from work lasting 4 or more weeks
d) Absences from work lasting 6 or more weeks
e) Absences from work lasting 5 or more years

QUESTION 45

A 35-year-old administrative assistant has been referred for advice managing her cancer. In your report you have stated that she should have time off for ongoing medical appointments. The manager is unclear about how they should proceed with this advice and asks you for guidance.

What is the most appropriate information you should give the manager regarding employee entitlement to time off for medical appointments?

a) Employees are legally entitled to paid time off for all medical appointments
b) Employees can take unpaid leave for medical appointments, but the employer must approve it

c) Employees do not have a legal right to paid or unpaid time off for routine medical appointments, unless stated in their contract
d) Employees are only entitled to time off for medical appointments if they have been employed for at least 12 months
e) Employees can take time off for medical appointments without needing to inform their employer in advance

QUESTION 46

You are asked to see a welder who is concerned about his risk of cancer from welding fumes after seeing an alert on TikTok.

What is the commonest type of cancer associated with welding fumes?

a) Bladder cancer
b) Melanoma
c) Prostate cancer
d) Renal carcinoma
e) Lung cancer

QUESTION 47

You are reviewing a pre-placement health questionnaire for an individual applying to work as a baker. The individual has a history of atopy.

What is the most appropriate next action you should take?

a) Fit for work
b) Fit for work with restrictions from working with asthmatogens
c) Unfit for work with asthmatogens
d) Fit for work as long as asthmatogen levels are ALARP
e) Fit for work with low molecular weight (LMW) asthmatogens only

QUESTION 48

You are implementing a screening programme for Covid-19 in a workplace. The Covid-19 test has a sensitivity of 90% and a specificity of 98%. You need to explain these statistics to the employer.

Which one of the following best explains the sensitivity of the Covid-19 test to the employer?

a) 90% of people with a Covid-19 infection will test positive on the test
b) 90% of people with a Covid-19 infection will test negative on the test
c) 90% of people without Covid-19 will test negative on the test
d) 90% of people who test positive on the test will actually have Covid-19
e) 90% of people who test negative on the test will not have Covid-19

QUESTION 49

You are asked to help set up the first aid provisions in a charity shop employing twenty people. You are asked to provide an opinion on the type of training needed for first aiders.

Which is the most likely training needed under the First Aid Regulations?

a) First aid at work
b) Emergency first aid at work
c) None – only an appointed person is needed
d) Mental health first aid
e) Paediatric first aid

QUESTION 50

A construction worker complains of symptoms suggestive of carpal tunnel syndrome (CTS) and on examination shows symptoms suggestive of sensorineural hand arm vibration syndrome (HAVS).

What is the most appropriate next step?

a) The severity of HAVS should be graded
b) Refer to a neurologist
c) Refer for further assessment of CTS
d) Refer for treatment of HAVS
e) Refer for Tier 5 assessment

QUESTION 51

A 58-year-old office worker has been on extended medical leave due to a chronic illness. The company has referred you to consider the employee for ill-health retirement under the company's pension scheme.

Which one of the following actions should the medical practitioner prioritise when assessing the employee's eligibility for an early retirement pension?

a) A review of the employee's current health status
b) A review of the previous occupational health reports to formulate an opinion
c) Writing to the employee's treating doctors to get the employee's medical history
d) Review the company pension scheme eligibility criteria
e) A review of the employee's sickness absence record

QUESTION 52

A manufacturing company conducts routine noise surveillance for its employees to monitor and protect their hearing health. The OH team is reviewing various methods and tests used in their programme.

Which one of the following is NOT part of routine noise surveillance?

a) Otoacoustic emission (OAE) tests
b) Questionnaire
c) Pure tone audiometry
d) Otoscopic examination
e) Health promotion

QUESTION 53

While conducting a training session for new employees on workplace health and safety measures, you describe the hierarchy of control.

Which of the following controls is considered the control of last resort?

a) Administrative
b) Elimination
c) Personal protective equipment (PPE)
d) Substitution
e) Engineering

QUESTION 54

A company that works with ionising radiation is conducting baseline medical surveillance to assess the fitness of its employees for their intended work.

Which of the following factors is most relevant to assess in detail when undertaking baseline health surveillance for work with ionising radiation (IR)?

a) Whether the employee has the physical dexterity to perform the role
b) Whether the employee has a history of neurological disease
c) Whether the employee has a history of cardiovascular disease
d) Whether the employee has a history of previous significant medical exposure to ionising radiation
e) All of the above

QUESTION 55

You are working with a large law firm to help them tender for a new OH provider. You are discussing the importance of accreditation and quality standards in OH services during a team meeting when an HR colleague asks about a specific accreditation standard that is widely recognised in the UK, SEQOHS.

What does SEQOHS stand for?

a) Safe Ethical Quality Occupational Health Service
b) Standardised Effective Qualified Occupational Health Service
c) Safe Effective Quality Occupational Health Service
d) Standardised Efficient Quality Occupational Health Service
e) Safe Effective Quantifiable Occupational Health Standards

QUESTION 56

As part of his pre-placement health screening of health workers you see a locum consultant who has come to the UK in the last year from a low-TB incidence country.

What is the most appropriate first step in his assessment to ensure he does not have tuberculosis (TB)?

a) Chest X-ray
b) Interferon-gamma test

c) Enquire about a personal or family history of TB
d) No further action: locums do not need further tests as they are not permanent staff
e) No further action: he has come from a low-TB incidence country

QUESTION 57

You are an OH specialist reviewing a study conducted to investigate the potential link between exposure to a hazardous chemical in the workplace and the development of a specific type of cancer. The study involved identifying workers who have already developed the cancer and a comparison group of workers who do not have the cancer. The investigators then looked back at their exposure histories to determine if there was a higher prevalence of exposure to the hazardous chemical among those who developed the cancer.

What type of study design best describes the method used in this investigation?

a) Prospective cohort study
b) Retrospective cohort study
c) Ecological study
d) Case–control study
e) Cross-sectional survey

QUESTION 58

A factory employs workers exposed to various hazardous substances, including lead and asbestos. Management is reviewing regulatory requirements for medical surveillance to ensure compliance.

Under which of the following regulations might medical surveillance by an appointed doctor be required?

a) Control of Noise at Work Regulations 2005
b) Control of Asbestos Regulations 2012
c) Manual Handling Operations Regulations 1992
d) Health and Safety (Display Screen Equipment) Regulations 1992
e) Control of Major Accident Hazards (COMAH) Regulations 2015

Questions and Answers for the Diploma in Occupational Medicine

QUESTION 59

You are assessing a 48-year-old lorry driver for a renewal of his licence with a diagnosis of angina. Whilst in the waiting room you notice that he needs to use his GTN spray.

In the consultation room you inform him that you cannot renew his licence as he has ongoing chest pain, and that he needs to inform the DVLA. He refuses to accept this and tells you that he needs to have his licence renewed or he will lose his job.

What is the most appropriate next step?

a) Arrange a cardiology follow-up for further investigation
b) Arrange a second opinion on his fitness to drive
c) Renew his licence
d) Speak to your defence union
e) Inform the DVLA

QUESTION 60

You are an OH professional conducting a risk assessment for a 35-year-old factory worker with managerial duties who has recently been diagnosed with epilepsy. The worker's seizures are currently not well-controlled, and you need to determine the appropriate work restrictions to ensure their safety.

Which of the following work activities is most appropriate to restrict for an employee with poorly-controlled epilepsy?

a) Clerical work at a desk with occasional computer use
b) Operating a hand-held power tool with an automatic shut-off feature
c) Supervising other workers while standing on the ground floor
d) Driving a forklift in a warehouse environment
e) Performing routine inventory checks in a storage room

QUESTION 61

As the senior OHP, you are approached by a new medical administrator in your department who is archiving old records. She seeks clarification on how long the clinical records of employees should be retained for. Her main concern is ensuring compliance with the specific regulatory requirements governing OH records.

For how long should these records be retained?

a) Keep the records for a period of 30 years following the last date of entry
b) Preserve the records until 100 years after the employee's birth date
c) Either until 6 years after retirement or until they reach 75 years of age, whichever is sooner
d) Retain the records indefinitely or until the individual dies
e) Until the employee's official retirement age as defined by employment contract

QUESTION 62

An office worker is about to undergo total hip replacement surgery and has been proactively referred for advice so that the team can plan for her absence.

According to guidance on returning to work after hip replacement surgery, which of the following is the most appropriate advice for an uncomplicated recovery?

a) They can return to work immediately after surgery as long as they are not experiencing pain and follow their surgeon's advice
b) They can typically return to work within 4–6 weeks if their job involves mostly sedentary activities and they follow their surgeon's advice
c) They can typically return to work within 12–24 weeks if their job involves mostly sedentary activities and they follow their surgeon's advice
d) They must wait at least 12 weeks before returning to any form of work, including sedentary tasks
e) They must wait at least 16 weeks before returning to any form of work, including sedentary tasks

QUESTION 63

A trainee nurse has sustained a high-risk needlestick injury. Management is seeking advice on any work restrictions that should be imposed during the follow-up testing period.

What is the best advice you should give management regarding restrictions on the trainee nurse during their follow-up tests?

a) They should be restricted from all clinical work until follow-up tests are complete
b) They should be restricted from performing exposure-prone procedures (EPPs) until follow-up tests are complete
c) They can continue to work without restrictions during the follow-up period
d) They should only be allowed to work in non-clinical areas until all test results are complete
e) They should be restricted from any work that could put them in contact with any bodily fluids until all test results are complete

QUESTION 64

You are giving a lecture about the risks of ultraviolet (UV) radiation.

In which one of the following occupations is there a statistically significant increased risk of ocular melanoma?

a) Construction workers
b) Airline pilots
c) Welders
d) Healthcare workers
e) Fishermen

QUESTION 65

You are teaching a group of medical students about the Equality Act 2010 and its role in protecting individuals from discrimination in the workplace and other settings.

Which one of the following is a protected characteristic under the Equality Act 2010?

a) Gender reassignment
b) Nationality

c) Socioeconomic status
d) Caring responsibilities
e) Employment status

QUESTION 66

You are evaluating the performance of a new diagnostic test for a workplace health surveillance programme. In a population of 1000 individuals, 100 are confirmed to have the disease based on a gold standard test. The new diagnostic test correctly identifies 80 individuals with the disease.

What is the sensitivity of the diagnostic test?

a) 4%
b) 10%
c) 40%
d) 80%
e) 90%

QUESTION 67

You are reviewing the spirometry results of a 55-year-old employee who presents for health surveillance with a history of chronic cough and shortness of breath.

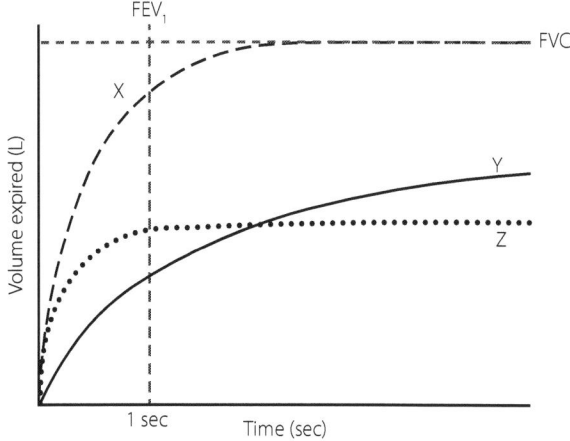

The spirometry is represented by line Y on the graph.

What is the most likely pathology?

a) Restrictive disease
b) Mixed obstructive and restrictive disease
c) Normal lung function
d) Abnormal lung function
e) Obstructive disease

QUESTION 68

You are conducting a training session on occupational toxicology for a group of new employees at a chemical manufacturing plant. During the session, you explain that understanding toxicokinetics is essential for assessing the potential health effects of chemical exposures.

What are the four components of toxicokinetics?

a) Absorption, Distribution, Metabolism, Excretion
b) Accumulation, Distribution, Diffusion, Excretion
c) Absorption, Digestion, Metabolism, Excretion
d) Accumulation, Distribution, Metabolism, Elimination
e) Absorption, Diffusion, Metabolism, Excretion

QUESTION 69

A junior health and safety officer reviewing workplace procedures for managing exposure to hazardous substances asks you where they can find the official workplace exposure limits (WELs) to ensure compliance with current regulations.

What is the most appropriate answer?

a) Google
b) *Oxford Handbook of Occupational Medicine*
c) EH40
d) RIDDOR
e) COSHH regulations

Questions for Mock exam 3

QUESTION 70

As part of your research project on occupational cancers in the UK, you are reviewing previous research on the industry with the highest incidence of occupational cancer cases.

Based on current evidence, which UK industry is known to have the highest burden of occupational cancers?

a) Agriculture
b) Construction
c) Manufacturing
d) Mining
e) Nuclear power

QUESTION 71

An employer is developing a strategy to manage dust exposure in the workplace and needs to understand the order of priority for implementing control measures to effectively reduce exposure to dust.

In managing dust exposure, which one of the following control measures should be prioritised?

a) Provide personal protective equipment (PPE) such as gloves, coveralls and a respirator
b) Apply administrative controls, such as reducing the length of time that workers are exposed to dust
c) Extract dust emissions near the source
d) Enclose the process so that dust does not escape
e) Minimise the number of workers that are at risk

QUESTION 72

You are assisting a large manufacturing company in updating its food handler policy. Management is looking for a precise definition of a 'food handler' to ensure the policy is clear and comprehensive.

What is the best definition of a 'food handler'?

a) A person who comes into direct contact with uncooked food at any point in the manufacturing process

b) A person who manufactures, prepares or transports food and may come into direct contact with food or with machines handling unwrapped food
c) Any person who works with cooked or uncooked food at any point in the manufacturing process
d) Any person who works in the food industry
e) A person who manages food inventory and ensures food is stored correctly

QUESTION 73

You are the OHP seeing an 18-year-old gardener who has exceeded her sickness absence threshold due to frequent absences from work. She has recently developed symptoms of seasonal allergic rhinitis during the spring and summer seasons. Her symptoms include frequent sneezing, itchy and watery eyes, and nasal congestion, which pose significant challenges for her while working outdoors in gardens with high pollen levels. Despite starting antihistamines recently, she has not experienced relief from her symptoms. She does not have any other medical conditions.

What is the most suitable advice to include in your report concerning the Equality Act 2010?

a) Seasonal allergic rhinitis is considered a disability under the Equality Act 2010 if medication is needed
b) Seasonal allergic rhinitis is covered as a disability under the Equality Act 2010 from diagnosis
c) Seasonal allergic rhinitis is covered as a disability under the Equality Act 2010 only if it requires ongoing medical treatment
d) Seasonal allergic rhinitis is not covered as a disability under the Equality Act 2010, except where it aggravates the effects of another condition
e) Seasonal allergic rhinitis is covered as a disability under the Equality Act if it is likely to recur over a period of twelve months or more

QUESTION 74

During a consultation, an employee undergoing her third round of *in vitro* fertilisation (IVF) treatment expresses frustration because her managers are not allowing her paid time off to attend IVF-related medical appointments. She mentions that this is causing conflict in the team, as pregnant employees are being given paid time off for antenatal appointments. The employee has been referred to you for work-related stress due to this situation.

What is the most appropriate response regarding the employee's rights to time off for IVF treatment?

a) The employee is legally entitled to paid time off for IVF treatment, similar to paid leave for antenatal appointments
b) There is no legal right to paid time off for IVF treatment, but the employer should be encouraged to treat this the same as any other medical appointment or sickness absence
c) The employee must use annual leave for IVF-related appointments, as there is no requirement for the employer to provide paid time off for these appointments
d) The employer is legally required to provide the same unpaid time off for IVF appointments as they do for antenatal appointments
e) The employee can request unpaid leave for IVF treatment, as it is not covered by any legal obligation for paid time off

QUESTION 75

During a training session for health and safety officers, you explain that certain exposures in the workplace contribute more significantly to cancer-related deaths than others. You highlight that, according to recent data, one substance is responsible for the highest number of occupational cancer deaths in the UK.

Which one of the following is the leading cause of occupational cancer deaths in Great Britain?

a) Diesel engine exhaust
b) Mineral oils
c) Shift work
d) Silica
e) Asbestos

QUESTION 76

You are an OHP undertaking an assessment of a 30-year-old industrial radiographer who has recently notified her employer that she is pregnant.

What is the most appropriate action the employer should take?

a) Make sure the pregnant employee's exposure is limited to ensure the foetal dose is unlikely to exceed 5 mSv during the remainder of the pregnancy

b) Allow the pregnant employee to continue work with radionuclides as long as proper personal protective equipment (PPE) is used
c) Make sure that the pregnant employee's work conditions are adjusted to ensure the foetal dose is unlikely to exceed 1 mSv during the remainder of the pregnancy
d) Permit the pregnant employee to continue her current duties without any modification, as long as her cumulative radiation dose has not yet reached the annual occupational limit
e) Transfer her to a role that does not involve exposure to ionising radiation for the remainder of her pregnancy

QUESTION 77

A worker has been diagnosed with a condition that may be reportable.

Which one of the following conditions is not classified as a reportable occupational disease under RIDDOR?

a) Carpal tunnel syndrome
b) Cramp of the hand or forearm
c) Occupational dermatitis
d) Noise-induced hearing loss
e) Hand arm vibration syndrome

QUESTION 78

You are seeing a 35-year-old factory worker with well-controlled insulin-dependent diabetes. He has been referred for advice on whether he can safely work rotating shifts, and he is eager to start as soon as possible.

What is the most appropriate advice for you to provide regarding his suitability for working on rotating shifts?

a) He should avoid rotating shifts entirely, as they are incompatible with insulin-dependent diabetes
b) He can start working rotating shifts but needs to undertake continuous glucose monitoring
c) He can work rotating shifts but may need to make adjustments to his meal schedule and glucose monitoring

d) He should work only fixed shifts to avoid potential risks of hypoglycaemia
e) He can work rotating shifts but cannot work alone due to the risk of hypoglycaemia

QUESTION 79

A 32-year-old office worker, who is 28 weeks pregnant, has been referred to you for advice on workplace adjustments. She has recently been started on insulin for gestational diabetes. She is under the care of both an obstetrician and an endocrinologist, and so far she has not experienced any disabling hypoglycaemic events, and is not expected to experience any. She is concerned about how her condition and insulin treatment might affect her ability to drive safely on her 20-minute commute to work.

What is the most appropriate advice regarding her driving while being treated with insulin?

a) She should stop driving immediately and notify the DVLA of her condition
b) She may continue driving and does not need to notify the DVLA
c) She should only drive after eating a meal and checking her blood glucose levels
d) She must notify the DVLA immediately due to the insulin treatment
e) She may continue driving but needs to notify the DVLA

QUESTION 80

You are reviewing the pre-placement questionnaire of a nurse who was born and raised in the UK and has applied for a role at the local hospital. The nurse has indicated that she had chickenpox at the age of 5.

What is the most appropriate next step?

a) Arrange an appointment to clarify the history of chickenpox
b) Arrange for varicella zoster virus (VZV) immunoglobulin to be administered
c) Clear her for non-clinical roles
d) No further action needed, she can be cleared to work
e) Serological testing

ANSWERS to Mock exam 3

QUESTION 1

You are leading an orientation session for new occupational health (OH) practitioners in a large industrial company. During the session, one of the practitioners asks about the legal framework that governs workplace safety and health.

Which of the following best describes the difference between an Act and a Regulation?

The answer is: b) An Act establishes the overall legal framework, while a Regulation is a detailed rule made under the Act to implement and enforce its provisions

An Act provides the broad legal structure that outlines employers' duties and employees' rights, while Regulations are specific rules under the Act that detail how to comply with those duties and enforce the standards necessary for workplace safety and health.

The specific rules are usually outlined in the Regulations, whereas the Act provides the general legal framework.

Both Acts and Regulations are legally binding, and compliance with both is mandatory in the workplace.

Both Acts and Regulations can be amended or repealed depending on legislative processes.

Source: www.legislation.gov.uk/understanding-legislation

QUESTION 2

You are advising an employer who is facing a conflict between medical opinions regarding an employee's fitness for work. The employee's GP has stated on the 'fit' note that the individual is unfit for work, while the OH professional has provided a robust report after gaining information from the employee's specialist indicating the employee is fit to return with reasonable adjustments. The employer is unsure which medical opinion to prioritise in making their decision.

What is the most reasonable action for the employer to take in this situation?

The answer is: c) Follow the recommendation of the OH professional, as tribunals typically consider this a reasonable approach

Employers may face conflicting medical opinions regarding an employee's fitness for work. Tribunals typically accept that a reasonable employer would rely on the advice of the OH, unless:
- the OH professional has not personally examined the employee
- the OH report is vague or inconclusive
- continued employment poses a significant health or safety risk to the individual or others
- the employee is under specialist care, and the OH professional has not consulted the specialist
- the employee requests to present an alternative specialist opinion.

Employers must ensure OH advice is thorough and well-documented to support their decisions.

Source: Hobson, J. and Smedley, J. (eds) (2019) *Fitness for Work: the medical aspects*, 6th edition. Oxford University Press

QUESTION 3

An occupational health physician (OHP) is evaluating an employee with a medical condition. The employer seeks clarification on whether the employee's condition meets the legal definition of disability under the Equality Act (EqA).

Which entity has the authority to make a final legal determination regarding whether an employee's condition satisfies the definition of disability under the EqA?

The answer is: c) The employment tribunal (ET)

Answers to Mock exam 3

The ET has the authority to make the final legal determination regarding whether an employee's condition qualifies as a disability under the Equality Act (EqA). While the OH professional, primary care physician and specialist physician can provide medical insights and evidence about the condition, it is the ET that evaluates whether the condition meets the legal criteria of having a substantial and long-term adverse effect on day-to-day activities, thus qualifying as a disability under the EqA.

Source: Hobson, J. and Smedley, J. (eds) (2019) *Fitness for Work: the medical aspects*, 6th edition. Oxford University Press

QUESTION 4

You are evaluating a 20-year-old warehouse operative who has just had his driver's licence revoked following a recent seizure. Prior to the recent seizure, he had been seizure-free for the past 10 years. Management is seeking advice on whether he is fit to undertake his role, which involves manual handling and forklift truck driving.

Which of the following options is the most appropriate advice regarding the fitness of the warehouse operative to undertake his role following the seizure?

The answer is: e) Restrict from forklift truck driving

Given the recent seizure, the operative should be restricted from forklift truck driving.

The immediate priority is to restrict him from activities that could pose a risk to himself and others if he were to have another seizure, particularly driving a forklift.

Source: Sadhra, S., Bray, A.J. and Boorman, S. (eds) (2022) *Oxford Handbook of Occupational Health*, third edition

QUESTION 5

You are consulting with a 55-year-old gardener who is seeking advice on returning to work after a total hip replacement. He is extremely worried that he will not be able to return to his job following the operation.

What percentage of individuals manage to return to their original work after a total hip replacement?

The answer is: c) 80–100% of patients manage to return to their original work

Following hip replacement surgery 80–100% of patients manage to return to their original work. Individual assessment helps. Some patients may require permanent relocation.

Source: Sadhra, S., Bray, A.J. and Boorman, S. (eds) (2022) *Oxford Handbook of Occupational Health*, third edition

QUESTION 6

You are reviewing the case of a healthcare worker (HCW) living with hepatitis B virus (HBV) who has been cleared to perform exposure-prone procedures (EPPs).

Who is primarily responsible for the ongoing monitoring of this HCW to ensure compliance with health and safety regulations?

The answer is: d) The accredited specialist in occupational medicine

The accredited specialist in occupational medicine is responsible for monitoring healthcare workers cleared to perform EPPs to ensure their fitness to continue performing these tasks safely.

The treating physician is responsible for providing care related to the HCW's blood-borne virus (BBV) infection, but not for occupational health clearance and monitoring related to EPPs.

Source: https://assets.publishing.service.gov.uk/media/6627a9b0d29479e036a7e622/integrated-guidance-for-management-of-BBV-in-HCW-April-2024-update.pdf

QUESTION 7

During a teaching session for medical students, you are asked a question about the role of an occupational hygienist. The students want to understand the primary responsibilities of an occupational hygienist within the workplace.

Which of the following best describes the primary role of an occupational hygienist?

The answer is: e) To identify, evaluate and manage work-related hazards that may contribute to employee health issues

The primary role of an occupational hygienist is to recognise, assess and control hazards in the workplace that could impact employees' health. This option accurately represents the focus of an occupational hygienist's responsibilities.

To design or modify the work to fit the worker: option a) describes the role of an ergonomist, who focuses on designing tasks, equipment and environments that accommodate workers' physical capabilities and limitations.

To apply psychology to the workplace to improve the effectiveness of organisations and the job satisfaction of employees: option b) describes the role of an occupational or organisational psychologist, who focuses on workplace morale and productivity, not on managing physical, chemical or biological hazards.

QUESTION 8

You are an OHP who has completed an assessment of a 40-year-old construction worker with chronic knee pain. The worker requested to see a copy of the report before it was sent to their employer. You provided the report to the worker and allowed a reasonable timeframe for them to review and provide feedback. Despite this, you have not received any response from the worker within the specified period.

What is the most appropriate next step in this situation?

The answer is: d) Assume the worker has no concerns and send the report to the employer without further action

While it is important to provide workers the opportunity to review and comment on their report, once a reasonable timeframe has been provided and no feedback is received, it is appropriate to proceed with sending the report to the employer. There is no requirement to obtain positive affirmation of consent or to delay the process further if the worker has not responded within the given timeframe. This approach ensures that the process remains efficient and timely, respecting the needs of both the worker and the employer.

Withdrawing the report due to lack of reaffirmation (option a) is unnecessary if a reasonable time has already been allowed for review.

Waiting an additional few weeks before taking any action to ensure the worker has sufficient time to respond could introduce unnecessary delays, especially if the initial timeframe was already reasonable.

While following up (option c) is a good practice, it may not be necessary if the initial period was adequate and a reminder might not be required.

Re-sending the report (option e) might be redundant if the worker was already given a reasonable opportunity to review it.

Source: www.fohn.org.uk/wp-content/uploads/2022/11/FOHN-Consent-and-Confidentiality-in-occupational-health.pdf

QUESTION 9

A sanitation worker presents for an occupational health assessment. He frequently works with raw, untreated sewage and asks about vaccination recommendations to protect his health.

Which of the following is the most appropriate preventive measure for workers exposed to raw sewage?

The answer is: c) Immunisation against hepatitis A

Sanitation workers frequently exposed to raw sewage are at increased risk of hepatitis A due to its transmission through contaminated water and sewage. Hepatitis A immunisation is recommended for those at risk of repeated exposure to untreated sewage to prevent infection. Other vaccines may be relevant depending on individual circumstances, but hepatitis A is the most directly related to this occupational exposure.

Source: https://assets.publishing.service.gov.uk/media/65a1743269fbd3000d25c075/Greenbook-chapter-17-hepatitis-A-12January24.pdf

QUESTION 10

You are part of a committee which has proposed a study to look at whether exposure to nanoparticles is linked to renal failure.

The proposed study methodology data is to be obtained from groups who have been exposed, or not exposed, to nanoparticles.

Which type of study does this best describe?

The answer is: d) Cohort study

A cohort study is an observational study comparing exposed vs. unexposed groups to study the effects of risk factors.

In a randomised controlled trial (RCT) participants are randomly assigned to treatment or control groups, to evaluate the effect of an intervention.

A case–control study compares patients with a disease (cases) to those without (controls), to assess exposure history.

A cross-sectional survey examines disease and other variables at a single time point. Best for prevalence studies.

In a crossover design each participant receives both treatments in sequence (e.g. A → B), suitable for reversible outcomes.

Source: www.cebm.ox.ac.uk/resources/ebm-tools/study-designs

QUESTION 11

Looking at the dose–response curves, which one of the following is correct?

The answer is: b) Y is the lowest observed level

V = threshold below which individual does not respond

W = mean toxic dose (MTD) or medial lethal dose, i.e. dose at which 50% of those exposed die

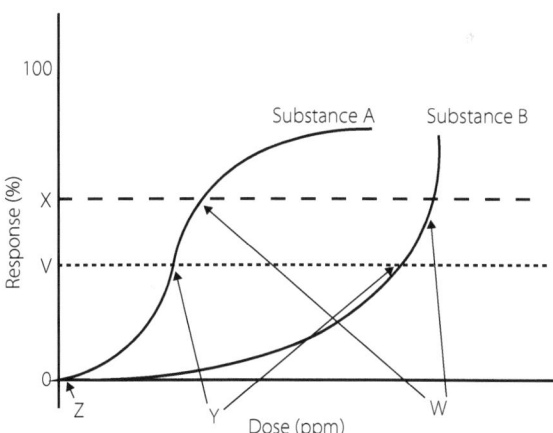

Note: ppm = parts per million

X = 50% response

Y = lowest observed effect level (LOEL), i.e. lowest dose at which effects occur

Z = no observed effect level (NOEL), i.e. at this level there are no observable effects

QUESTION 12

You are the occupational physician in a large company that makes furniture. There is poor compliance with controls and you are concerned about the employees' exposure to wood dust.

Which of the following is most associated with wood dust exposure?

The answer is: c) Sinonasal carcinoma

Long-term exposure to wood dust, a known risk factor for sinonasal carcinoma, makes this type of cancer the most likely diagnosis. Sinonasal carcinoma is specifically associated with occupational wood dust exposure. The other cancers listed are not commonly linked with wood dust exposure.

Source: https://assets.publishing.service.gov.uk/media/5a81bd1c40f0b 62302698e58/print-ready-nasal-carcinoma-and-occupational-exposure-to-wood-dust-iiac-report.pdf

QUESTION 13

A 50-year-old female textile worker presents to the clinic with complaints of chest tightness, coughing, wheezing and shortness of breath that began a few months ago. She reports that these symptoms are most severe at the beginning of the work week and gradually improve by the end of the week. She notices significant relief from her symptoms during weekends and vacations when she is away from work. The patient has worked in a textile factory for the past 20 years. She has a history of smoking 10 cigarettes a day since the age of 20 but has no other known medical problems. Spirometry shows a reduced FEV_1.

What is the most likely diagnosis?

The answer is: b) Byssinosis

Byssinosis, also known as 'Monday fever', is the most likely diagnosis in this scenario. It is an occupational lung disease seen in textile workers due to exposure to cotton dust. The hallmark of byssinosis is the pattern of symptoms that are worse at the beginning of the work week and improve by the end of the week or when the worker is away from the workplace. The patient's work history, symptom pattern and reduced FEV_1 on spirometry support this diagnosis.

Although occupational asthma can present with symptoms such as chest tightness, coughing, wheezing and shortness of breath, it typically does not show the pattern of symptom fluctuation that is strongly tied to the beginning of the work week and improvement over the weekend. Occupational asthma symptoms would generally persist as long as the worker is exposed to the causative agent.

While COPD could explain some of the patient's respiratory symptoms and reduced FEV_1, it does not typically exhibit a pattern where symptoms fluctuate based on the work week. Additionally, COPD symptoms usually worsen progressively over time and are more constant rather than improving when the patient is away from work. This makes COPD less likely than byssinosis, given the specific context of occupational exposure and symptom fluctuation.

Hypersensitivity pneumonitis can present with respiratory symptoms due to exposure to inhaled organic dusts, but it generally causes more chronic and persistent symptoms. It also typically presents with more systemic symptoms such as fever and malaise.

Tuberculosis (TB) is a chronic infectious disease that would present with more persistent symptoms, such as a chronic cough, night sweats, weight loss and potentially haemoptysis, rather than a pattern of symptoms that worsen during the work week and improve on weekends. Additionally, TB would not be expected to cause a decrease in FEV_1 related to workplace exposure, further ruling it out in favour of byssinosis.

Source: www.mountsinai.org/health-library/diseases-conditions/byssinosis#:~:text=It%20is%20most%20common%20in,still%20common%20in%20developing%20countries

QUESTION 14

A surgeon has been diagnosed with dry age-related macular degeneration which has become significantly worse over the last 5 months.

For this reason, their employer reviews the situation and decides they need to stop the surgeon performing operations.

The surgeon feels they are being discriminated against.

Which of the following is the best term for this?

The answer is: c) Objective justification

The employer decides to stop the surgeon from performing operations due to safety concerns for patients and the surgeon themself. This action, though seemingly discriminatory based on a disability, serves a legitimate aim of ensuring safety and is proportionate, appropriate and necessary. Thus, it falls under objective justification rather than direct discrimination or other forms of discriminatory actions listed.

An employer might need to make certain decisions that lead to discrimination. This might be legal if there is 'objective justification'.

Under the law, there can be objective justification if the employer can prove both of the following:
- There is a "legitimate aim" such as a genuine business need or a health and safety need
- The discrimination is "proportionate, appropriate and necessary" – this means the legitimate aim is more important than any discriminatory effect.

Employers are advised to consider less discriminatory alternatives and seek legal advice if uncertain.

Source: www.acas.org.uk/employer-decision-protected-characteristic/objective-justification

QUESTION 15

You are conducting a remote consultation with a 54-year-old man who recently experienced an uncomplicated cerebrovascular event while abroad on business. The man wishes to return home to his family, and his employer is seeking guidance on when he can safely travel by air.

What is the most appropriate advice regarding air travel following an uncomplicated cerebrovascular event?

The answer is: a) Air travel is contraindicated for at least 3 days after an uncomplicated cerebrovascular event

A recent cardiovascular event should result in caution because of the relative hypoxia and risk of a further acute event. As a general guide, do not allow air travel if myocardial infarct within 10 days if uncomplicated (3–4 weeks with complications), coronary angioplasty within 3–5 days, or cerebrovascular event within 3 days.

Sources:
- www.caa.co.uk/passengers-and-public/before-you-fly/am-i-fit-to-fly/guidance-for-health-professionals/cardiovascular-disease
- Sadhra, S., Bray, A.J. and Boorman, S. (eds) (2022) *Oxford Handbook of Occupational Health*, third edition

QUESTION 16

You are evaluating a 36-year-old construction worker who has been escalated to Tier 4 vibration health surveillance. He presents with sensory disturbances in the little and ring fingers, clawing of the hand, and atrophy of the hypothenar eminence. The fixed flexion test is positive.

What is the most likely diagnosis?

The answer is: b) Cubital tunnel syndrome

The symptoms described – sensory disturbances in the little and ring fingers, clawing of the hand, atrophy of the hypothenar eminence, and a positive fixed flexion test – are indicative of cubital tunnel syndrome.

QUESTION 17

An individual who is self-employed has sustained a work-related injury and is considering applying for Industrial Injuries Disablement Benefit (IIDB) and asks you about it.

Based on the eligibility criteria, which one of the following statements is correct?

The answer is: b) The individual cannot apply for IIDB because self-employed individuals are not eligible for this benefit

IIDB is specifically designed for employees who suffer from work-related injuries or diseases. Self-employed individuals are not eligible for IIDB, regardless of their work-related circumstances.

Apprenticeship status does not affect eligibility for IIDB.

While IIDB claims are generally related to the current or recent work, the key eligibility factor is that the claimant must be an employee at the time of application. The individual's employment status as self-employed or an employee is the critical issue; changing industries does not affect eligibility for IIDB.

Eligibility for IIDB does not require that the individual is currently working. The key requirement is that the person must have been an employee at the time the injury or illness occurred. If they were an employee at the time of the injury, they can still claim IIDB even if they are no longer working.

IIDB eligibility is not contingent on the individual's current employment status or industry. The primary criterion is that the individual must have been an employee at the time of the injury or illness. The industry relevance is not a factor in determining IIDB eligibility.

Source: www.gov.uk/industrial-injuries-disablement-benefit/eligibility

QUESTION 18

You undertake a workplace visit at a material recovery facility. It appears to be noisy, but no hygiene measurements are available. The noise appears intrusive, but normal conversation is possible. The supervisor informs you that the noise level is like this for the full 6-hour shift.

What would you estimate the noise level to be in your report?

The answer is: a) 80 dB(A)

A risk assessment is mandatory if any employee is likely to be exposed to noise at or above the lower exposure action value (EAV). Specifically, working in an environment with a noise level of 80 dB(A) for eight hours will reach this lower EAV.

The Health and Safety Executive (HSE) provides a basic system in the absence of formal dosimetry to estimate if a risk assessment is necessary based on the duration and intensity of noise exposure:
- 80 dB(A): if the noise is intrusive but normal conversation is possible, a risk assessment is needed if exposure is for more than 6 hours
- 85 dB(A): if you have to shout to talk to someone 2 metres away, a risk assessment is needed if exposure is for more than 2 hours
- 90 dB(A): if you have to shout to talk to someone 1 metre away, a risk assessment is needed if exposure is for more than 45 minutes.

Source: www.hse.gov.uk/pubns/priced/l108.pdf

QUESTION 19

You are delivering a lecture on screening tests and their effectiveness in OH settings. A trainee asks about the factors that influence the positive predictive value (PPV) of a test.

Which one of the following statements about the PPV of a screening test is correct?

The answer is: b) PPV increases with increasing sensitivity of the screening test

The positive predictive value (PPV) is the proportion of people who test positive on a diagnostic test who actually have the disease. While sensitivity and specificity are often described as constant characteristics of any screening test, the PPV of a test will vary with the population in which the test is being applied. If the disease prevalence is low in the population tested, there will be a greater likelihood of false positive results, so that a given positive test has a low PPV.

PPV increases with increasing disease prevalence.

PPV increases with increasing sensitivity of the screening test.

PPV decreases for a rare disease, but increases for a common disease with increasing specificity of the screening test.

Source: Hobson, J. and Smedley, J. (eds) (2019) *Fitness for Work: the medical aspects*, 6th edition. Oxford University Press

QUESTION 20

You are an OHP conducting a telephone consultation with Mr Patel, a 40-year-old employee seeking advice on managing stress-related symptoms at work. Mr Patel has signed the consent form sent with the referral to take part in the consultation.

What is the best practice for taking consent in remote occupational health consultations?

The answer is: e) Record Mr Patel's verbal consent in the consultation notes contemporaneously

In remote OH consultations, verbal consent is often obtained due to the nature of the interaction. This includes reaffirming signed consent prior to the consultation. It is crucial to document this consent immediately in the consultation notes. This documentation should include specific details such as Mr Patel's agreement to proceed with the assessment, understanding of the purpose of the consultation, and acknowledgment of what information will be included in the report. This approach ensures transparency and compliance with data protection regulations.

While an email confirmation (prior to or post-consultation) can be a form of documentation, it may not capture real-time consent during the consultation itself. Verbal consent documented contemporaneously is preferable for ensuring clarity and immediacy in understanding Mr Patel's agreement.

Assuming implicit consent without explicit confirmation during the session does not align with best practices for informed consent in occupational health. Contemporary verbal or documented consent is necessary to ensure Mr Patel fully understands and agrees to the consultation process.

Source: www.fohn.org.uk/wp-content/uploads/2022/11/FOHN-Consent-and-Confidentiality-in-occupational-health.pdf

QUESTION 21

Dr Grimes, an OH consultant, has been asked to review the devised plan for a new out-of-hours service at a large hospital. The goal is to ensure that the new shift patterns are safe and effective for both staff and patients. The current plan includes forward rotating shifts, timing shifts to avoid starting before 7am, limiting shift duration to 12 hours, providing adequate rest breaks, and ensuring compliance with the Working Time Regulations 1998.

Based on the principles of effective shift design, what is the most appropriate recommendation for Dr Grimes to make?

The answer is: b) Consider lighting and temperature adjustments during night shifts

Ensuring proper lighting and temperature for night shifts is crucial for maintaining safety and comfort, which helps to mitigate the adverse effects of working overnight. Adequate lighting ensures work can be performed safely, while maintaining a comfortable temperature helps manage the natural drop in body temperature overnight.

Allowing staff to sleep on site after an 11-hour shift, while potentially beneficial for rest, is impractical.

Mandating staff not to exceed shift length and ensuring compliance with regulations is important, but it is sometimes impractical due to emergencies on shift.

Monitoring and recording shift swapping is crucial for ensuring necessary rest periods and avoiding excessive hours, contributing to staff wellbeing and compliance with regulations, but banning staff from swapping shifts is impractical.

Providing vending machines with affordable food options supports staff health and wellbeing, but it is not a core element of effective shift design.

Source: www.nhsemployers.org/system/files/media/Supporting-the-wellbeing-of-shiftworkers-in-healthcare_0.pdf

QUESTION 22

You are providing a training session for managers on employer responsibilities and their duty of care to their employees. During the session, you explain the 'eggshell skull' principle.

Which one of the following does the 'eggshell skull' principle imply for employers?

The answer is: c) Employers owe a higher duty of care to employees with known vulnerabilities

Employers must exercise greater care for employees with pre-existing medical conditions or vulnerabilities, as outlined by the 'eggshell skull' principle. This is because they are deemed more vulnerable to injury than those of good health. Therefore, it is important that employers seek expert occupational health advice on fitness for work, job placements, and any special measures required to fulfil these obligations and reduce legal risks.

Source: Hobson, J. and Smedley, J. (eds) (2019) *Fitness for Work: the medical aspects*, 6th edition. Oxford University Press

QUESTION 23

An occupational hygienist is measuring sound levels in a workplace to assess potential hearing risks. The professional explains that the human ear is more sensitive to certain frequencies than others, and sound measurements should consider this sensitivity to obtain accurate readings.

When measuring sound levels in the workplace to evaluate potential hearing risks, which weighting should be used?

The answer is: d) A-weighting

The most commonly used weighting is the A-weighting because it mimics the response of the human ear. The C-weighting should be applied when measuring the peak sound pressure level.

Source: Sadhra, S., Bray, A.J. and Boorman, S. (eds) (2022) *Oxford Handbook of Occupational Health*, third edition

QUESTION 24

You are asked to advise a group of engineers who work with rosin flux based on a review of a recently performed risk assessment.

Occupational hygiene measurements show that the time-weighted average (TWA) (8h) is 0.04 mg/m^3

Workplace exposure limit (WEL): 8h TWA rosin = 0.05 mg/m^3

Which one of the following is the most appropriate next step, based on the hygiene result, to mitigate the risk?

The answer is: b) Exposure should be reduced to the lowest level reasonably practicable

Even though the measured exposure (0.04 mg/m^3) is below the WEL (0.05 mg/m^3), it is still prudent to reduce exposure to the lowest level reasonably practicable. This approach follows the principle of ALARP (as low as reasonably practicable), which aims to minimise risks further where possible. Reducing exposure can provide a safety margin, cater for any variations in exposure, and account for any potential long-term health effects that may not be entirely mitigated by merely meeting the WEL.

Once this has been achieved, the next step in controlling the risk is to provide additional training and information to workers.

It is essential to continue periodic monitoring and review of the control measures once in place. This ensures that the control measures remain effective over time and that exposure does not increase due to changes in work practices, production rates or equipment degradation. Regular reviews also help identify any new potential risks and ensure ongoing compliance with occupational health standards.

Despite being below the WEL, COSHH mandates that asthmatogens must be kept below the WEL but more importantly ALARP.

Health surveillance is not a control, but can help detect early signs of adverse health effects among workers exposed to rosin flux, even at levels below the WEL. This proactive measure can lead to early intervention, preventing more severe health outcomes. Surveillance can include regular medical check-ups, respiratory function tests and skin examinations, as rosin flux can cause respiratory and dermal issues.

QUESTION 25

Mr Hassan was referred for fitness to attend a disciplinary. He had no underlying medical concerns. You discussed the importance of meeting with the employer to resolve the issue as soon as possible, as delay could actually cause more harm. Mr Hassan agreed to this and consented to the report being sent to HR. He also said he wanted to see the report before it was sent, and gave you an email address to use. You advised that when he received the report, he would have 48 hours in which to respond. Mr Hassan did not respond to OH or make any comment on the report within the 48-hour time period.

What is the most appropriate next step?

The answer is: a) Send the report to HR on the basis of the consent given during the consultation

The Faculty of Occupational Medicine recommends that you wait a specified amount of time (e.g. 2–3 days), and once this has elapsed then the report can be sent to management, on the basis that consent for the report was given during the consultation and has not been withdrawn.

Mr Hassan explicitly consented to the report being sent to HR during the consultation. The requirement to review the report was additional to this consent, not a precondition for it. Mr Hassan was given 48 hours to respond, which he did not. The failure to respond does not negate the initial consent given.

Therefore, sending the report to HR on the basis of the consent given during the consultation is the most appropriate next step.

Source: www.fohn.org.uk/wp-content/uploads/2022/11/FOHN-Consent-and-Confidentiality-in-occupational-health.pdf

QUESTION 26

You are conducting a workshop on disability discrimination for a group of Human Resources professionals. During the session, a question arises about whether an individual who has recovered from a health condition can still be considered disabled under the Equality Act 2010.

Which one of the following statements is true regarding the classification of a person as disabled under the Equality Act 2010?

The answer is: b) A person who has recovered can still be classified as disabled if all criteria for disability are met and the condition existed after the Equality Act 2010 came into effect

Under the Equality Act 2010, a person can still be classified as disabled if they have a history of a condition that meets the criteria for disability, even if they have since recovered. This retrospective classification is essential for addressing cases of discrimination based on past disabilities. However, for the classification to be valid, all criteria of disability under the Act must be met, and the condition must have existed since the legislation came into effect in 2010.

Source: www.equalityhumanrights.com/equality/equality-act-2010/your-rights-under-equality-act-2010/disability-discrimination

QUESTION 27

You are assessing a worker with a history of prolonged use of vibrating hand tools and symptoms suggestive of hand arm vibration syndrome (HAVS).

Answers to Mock exam 3

What grading system is commonly used to evaluate the severity of vascular and sensorineural deficits in HAVS?

The answer is: c) Stockholm Workshop Scale

The Stockholm Workshop Scale is the grading system used to evaluate the severity of vascular and sensorineural deficits in HAVS. It provides a structured approach to assess the extent of symptoms and their impact.

The Epworth score is used to assess daytime sleepiness.

International consensus score: while there is an international consensus on HAVS, this specific score is not commonly used to evaluate HAVS severity.

The Glasgow Coma Scale is used to assess the level of consciousness in patients with brain injury.

The Disabilities of the Arm, Shoulder, and Hand (DASH) score assesses upper extremity disability and symptoms.

Source: www.som.org.uk/sites/som.org.uk/files/HAVS_staging_guide_July_2022.pdf

QUESTION 28

You are reviewing the viral load results of an obstetrician who is HIV positive under your care. The viral load is reported as 2000 copies/ml.

What is the most appropriate next action?

The answer is: b) Restrict the obstetrician from performing EPPs with immediate effect

For healthcare workers (HCWs) performing exposure-prone procedures (EPPs), a viral load above 1000 copies/ml requires immediate restriction from EPPs. The HCW may only resume EPPs once their viral load is consistently below 200 copies/ml.

Source: Sadhra, S., Bray, A.J. and Boorman, S. (eds) (2022) *Oxford Handbook of Occupational Health*, third edition

QUESTION 29

You speak to a manager who wants to refer an individual who is neurodifferent for advice on adjustments.

What is the most common functional impairment in neurodifferent individuals?

The answer is: c) Memory/concentration

The Society of Occupational Medicine's *Evaluating and Supporting Neurodifferences at Work* states that the following areas of difficulty are typical for neurodifferent (ND) employees:
- Memory/concentration (>90% of ND employees experience this)
- Organisation and time management (>75% of ND employees)
- Managing stress (>65%)
- Communicating (>65%), which can include written communication accuracy and written communication speed

Source: www.som.org.uk/sites/som.org.uk/files/Evaluating_and_supporting_Neurodifferences_at_work_March_2022.pdf

QUESTION 30

You see a 65-year-old electrician referred with work-related stress. He tells you that he thinks his employer wants him to retire.

Which one of the following statements is accurate regarding retirement age?

The answer is: d) There is no mandatory age of retirement

Since 2011, the statutory default retirement age of 65 was abolished in the UK, meaning there is no mandatory retirement age. Employers cannot force employees to retire based solely on age, unless they can provide a justifiable reason for doing so.

Source: Sadhra, S., Bray, A.J. and Boorman, S. (eds) (2022) *Oxford Handbook of Occupational Health*, third edition

QUESTION 31

You are teaching a group of students about the principles of radiological protection. A student wants clarification about the effect of distance on radiation intensity.

What is the effect if you double the distance from the source of radiation?

The answer is: c) The radiation intensity is reduced to one-fourth

Radiation follows the inverse square law, that the intensity of radiation exposure is inversely proportional to the square of the distance from the source.

The principles of radiation protection (which aim to minimise occupational radiation exposure), describe the use of distance and the inverse square law to keep occupational exposure as low as reasonably practicable (ALARP).

The principles are:
- *Time*: limit the time spent in radiation areas to reduce exposure
- *Distance*: increase the distance from the radiation source, as exposure decreases with the square of the distance
- *Shielding*: use barriers, such as thick walls or lead shields, to block radiation and reduce exposure
- *Containment*: radioactive materials may be used in 'sealed sources' to prevent them spreading.

Source: https://hps.org/publicinformation/ate/faqs/radiation.html

QUESTION 32

A 45-year-old factory worker is undergoing routine health screening as part of an OH assessment. The company uses two different tests to screen for a common industrial disease. One test is known for its high sensitivity, the other test is noted for its high specificity.

Which of the following best describes the role of sensitivity and specificity in occupational health screening?

The answer is: b) Sensitivity is the ability to correctly identify workers who have the disease, while specificity is the ability to correctly identify workers who do not have the disease

Sensitivity is the ability to correctly identify workers who have the disease (true positives), while specificity is the ability to correctly identify workers who do not have the disease (true negatives). This distinction is crucial for determining which test to use for effective screening.

Source: https://blogs.imperial.ac.uk/medical-centre/2023/10/10/making-sense-of-sensitivity-specificity-and-predictive-value-a-guide-for-patients-clinicians-and-policymakers

QUESTION 33

A factory worker who recently moved to your area presents to your clinic with a history of stannosis. This condition was diagnosed in his previous job where he was exposed to dust.

Which one of the following causes stannosis?

The answer is: a) Tin dust

Stannosis is a rare form of pneumoconiosis caused by the inhalation of tin dust or tin oxide fumes.

QUESTION 34

You are undertaking a complex ill-health retirement case in which a 55-year-old employee has been absent from work for one year with fibromyalgia. The clinician is considering supporting ill-health retirement but wants to ensure the decision is based on the highest quality evidence available.

Which of the following represents the highest level of evidence to guide your decision?

The answer is: d) Systematic reviews

The hierarchy of evidence refers to a system used to rank research studies based on their methodological quality and ability to answer clinical or research questions. It is crucial for guiding evidence-based decision-making, ensuring the reliability and applicability of findings in healthcare and scientific practices.

This framework underpins systematic reviews and evidence-based practice.
1. Systematic reviews and meta-analyses
   - Synthesised analyses of multiple high-quality studies addressing the same research question
   - Offer the strongest evidence due to their methodological rigour and large sample sizes
   - Example: Cochrane Reviews.
2. Randomised controlled trials (RCTs)
   - Studies where participants are randomly assigned to intervention or control groups.

3. Cohort studies
   - Observational studies that follow groups with and without exposure to a risk factor over time
   - Provide data on the association between exposures and outcomes.
4. Case–control studies
   - Retrospective studies comparing individuals with a specific outcome (cases) to those without (controls)
   - Useful for studying rare conditions or diseases.
5. Cross-sectional studies and surveys
   - Studies that analyse data from a population at a single point in time
   - Suitable for understanding prevalence and associations but limited in causality.
6. Case reports and case series
   - Detailed reports of individual or grouped cases
   - Valuable for rare or novel conditions but lack generalisability.
7. Expert opinion and background information
   - Based on clinical expertise or foundational knowledge
   - Lowest level of evidence due to lack of systematic analysis.

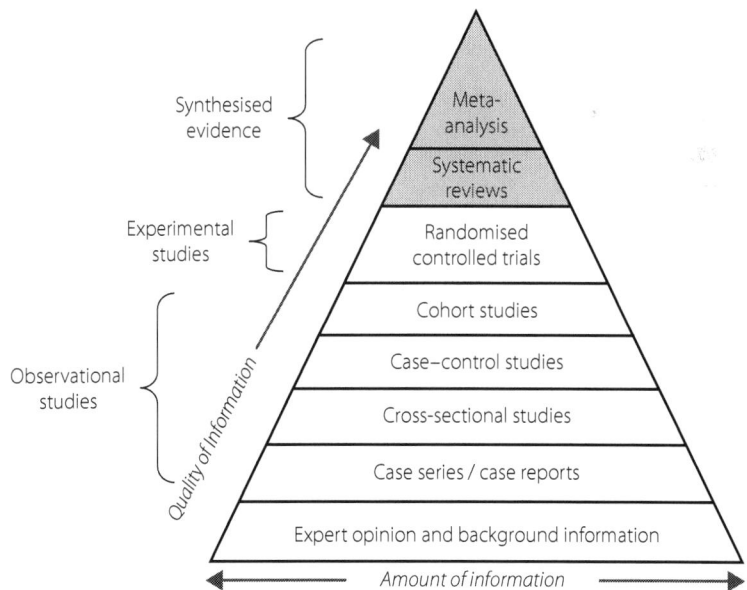

Source: https://guides.library.ucdavis.edu/systematic-reviews/levels-of-evidence

QUESTION 35

You are advising an employer about the increased vulnerabilities of young workers.

Which of the following would be considered a young worker?

The answer is: c) An individual aged under 18

The Management of Health and Safety at Work Regulations 1999 include specific measures to protect young people, defined as individuals under 18, in the workplace. These regulations recognise young workers' increased vulnerability due to limited work experience and potential physical or psychological immaturity.

Source: Sadhra, S., Bray, A.J. and Boorman, S. (eds) (2022) *Oxford Handbook of Occupational Health*, third edition

QUESTION 36

You are assisting an employer in setting up a drug and alcohol screening process for employees in safety-critical roles. A manager asks about the importance of a "chain of custody" in this context.

Which of the following best describes "chain of custody"?

The answer is: c) The process for managing the collection, handling, storage and testing of samples

"Chain of custody" refers to a strict protocol used to collect, handle and document drug and alcohol test samples to ensure their security and integrity throughout the testing process. This procedure ensures that samples are correctly labelled, securely stored, and accurately tracked from collection through testing to avoid contamination, tampering or mix-ups.

Source: Sadhra, S., Bray, A.J. and Boorman, S. (eds) (2022) *Oxford Handbook of Occupational Health*, third edition

QUESTION 37

A 52-year-old bus driver is diagnosed with a medical condition that may impact his ability to drive safely.

Which one of the following has the duty to inform the Driver and Vehicle Licensing Agency (DVLA)?

The answer is: e) Licence holder

In the UK, it is the legal responsibility of the licence holder to inform the DVLA of any medical condition or change in their health that may impact their fitness to drive. Although employers, GPs, specialists and OH professionals can advise and support the driver in this process, the duty to notify the DVLA lies with the individual driver.

Source: Sadhra, S., Bray, A.J. and Boorman, S. (eds) (2022) *Oxford Handbook of Occupational Health*, third edition

QUESTION 38

A 25-year-old chef has experienced three episodes of diarrhoea and has informed his manager, who then seeks your advice in advance to manage the chef's return to work.

What is the most appropriate response to give?

The answer is: c) He can return to work 48 hours after his symptoms stop

Guidelines, especially in food service, recommend that individuals should not return to work until at least 48 hours after symptoms (such as diarrhoea) have fully resolved. This helps ensure that the individual is no longer contagious and reduces the risk of spreading infection.

Diarrhoea can be highly contagious, and continuing to work could pose a significant health risk to colleagues and customers. Increased hand hygiene is important but insufficient to prevent the spread of infectious agents in a food-handling environment.

The recommendation is not based on when symptoms start. Allowing a return to work after a fixed period from the start of symptoms can still pose a risk of spreading infection, as the individual might still be symptomatic or contagious.

While medical clearance can be important in some contexts, it is generally not a standard requirement for returning to work after a typical bout of diarrhoea, provided that the symptoms have resolved for 48 hours.

Source: www.food.gov.uk/sites/default/files/media/document/fitnesstoworkguide.pdf

QUESTION 39

A receptionist in the emergency department was bitten by a patient known to be infected with hepatitis B. She is anxious about the risk of transmission and asks about the effectiveness of the hepatitis B vaccination course she started within the appropriate timeframe.

What is the effectiveness of the hepatitis B vaccination in preventing hepatitis B infection when given as post-exposure prophylaxis?

The answer is: d) >95%

A full vaccination course of hepatitis B, particularly when given within 24 hours but up to 7 days after exposure, is highly effective in preventing HBV infection, with an estimated effectiveness of over 95%. This estimate is based on extrapolated data from infant vaccination following birth exposure to hepatitis B. Post-exposure prophylaxis with the vaccine provides long-term protection and has a good safety profile, making it an effective method for preventing transmission after potential exposure.

Source: https://assets.publishing.service.gov.uk/media/5d948c36e5274a2fb1019c1a/Guidance_on_management_of_potential_exposure_to_blood__2_.pdf

QUESTION 40

A 55-year-old worker presents to the OH clinic for health surveillance. Spirometry is performed and the flow-volume loop shown below is observed.

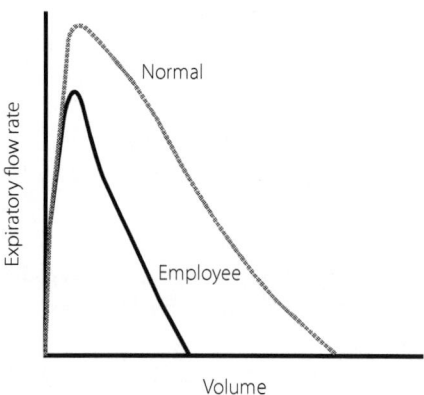

Which occupational hazard is most likely to cause the pulmonary function result shown?

The answer is: a) Silica

Silica exposure, especially in industries such as mining, construction and sandblasting, can lead to silicosis, a form of pneumoconiosis that is characterised by a restrictive lung disease pattern.

Flour dust is commonly associated with occupational asthma, leading to an obstructive rather than restrictive pattern.

Arsine is a gas that can cause haemolysis and acute toxicity but is not typically linked with chronic lung disease or a restrictive pattern.

Benzene is a well-known industrial chemical that is more commonly associated with haematologic disorders, such as leukaemia, rather than lung disease.

Rosin is primarily associated with allergic contact dermatitis and respiratory conditions such as asthma, which typically result in an obstructive pattern.

Source: www.brit-thoracic.org.uk/media/70454/spirometry_e-guide_2013.pdf

QUESTION 41

You are reviewing the occupational health risks associated with air conditioning engineers.

Which one of the following pathogens are air conditioning engineers more likely to be exposed to than the general population, due to their occupation?

The answer is: d) *Legionella pneumophila*

Air conditioning engineers are at an increased risk of *Legionella pneumophila* infection, which causes legionnaires' disease. This is due to their exposure to water systems, cooling towers and air conditioning units, which can harbour the *Legionella* bacterium. Contaminated water droplets dispersed through air conditioning systems can be inhaled, leading to infection. Proper maintenance and disinfection of these systems are essential to reduce this occupational health risk. The other infections listed are not typically associated with air conditioning work.

QUESTION 42

You are part of a working group discussing the potential classification of osteoarthritis as a prescribed disease in a platinum extraction process due to exposure to substance 'X' at the Industrial Injuries Advisory Council (IIAC).

The evidence does not appear clear-cut and the group is looking at any evidence of an increased relative risk of the disease in the occupational group.

What evidence of increased relative risk is needed to support the designation of a prescribed disease?

The answer is: b) More than 2

The law provides for payment of benefits to people who are suffering from certain diseases contracted in the course of certain types of employment. These diseases are referred to as prescribed diseases (PDs).

The IIAC is an independent scientific advisory body that looks at industrial injuries benefit and how it is administered.

When evaluating whether a disease should be designated as a PD, the IIAC looks for evidence that the disease is associated with a particular occupation. The IIAC normally seeks evidence that the 'relative risk' (RR) in a particular job with a particular exposure is more than 2.

A relative risk of more than 2 means that people who work in a particular type of job or who are exposed to a particular hazard at work are more than twice as likely to develop a particular disease as members of the general public who do not work in that type of job and are not exposed to that hazard but are in other ways the same. To put it another way, the risk of the disease is doubled for those working in that type of job or exposed to that hazard at work.

Source: https://assets.publishing.service.gov.uk/media/5a80c16040f0b 62302695526/iiac--iidb-prescribed-disease-decisions-faq-july-2015.pdf

QUESTION 43

You have started as the OP at a toothpaste factory and your first task is to help the business determine their first aid requirements. The factory employs 200 people.

What is the minimum number of first aiders needed in this factory?

The answer is: b) 4

Toothpaste manufacturing would fall under the high hazard category due to the potential use of machinery and chemicals in the production process.

For high hazard workplaces with more than 50 employees, the recommendation is at least 1 first aid at work trained first aider for every 50 employees or part thereof.

Calculation:

200 employees ÷ 50 employees per first aider = 4 first aiders.

Source: www.hse.gov.uk/pubns/priced/l74.pdf

QUESTION 44

A company is reviewing its policies on managing employee sickness absence. It is referring to guidelines from the National Institute for Health and Care Excellence (NICE) to determine what constitutes long-term sickness absence.

According to NICE, how is long-term sickness absence defined?

The answer is: c) Absences from work lasting 4 or more weeks

NICE defines long-term sickness absence as absences lasting 4 or more weeks.

For employees whose sickness absence is expected to extend beyond 4 weeks, organisations with occupational health providers should:
- discuss the option of referring the employee to occupational health for a fitness-for-work assessment
- consider early referral to support services if appropriate, and ensure that the referral occurs as soon as possible.

Source: www.nice.org.uk/guidance/ng146

QUESTION 45

A 35-year-old administrative assistant has been referred for advice managing her cancer. In your report you have stated that she should have time off for ongoing medical appointments. The manager is unclear about how they should proceed with this advice and asks you for guidance.

What is the most appropriate information you should give the manager regarding employee entitlement to time off for medical appointments?

The answer is: c) Employees do not have a legal right to paid or unpaid time off for routine medical appointments, unless stated in their contract

Employees do not have an automatic legal right to take paid or unpaid time off for routine medical appointments, unless this is specifically provided for in their employment contract or company policy. It is important for employees to check their contracts or speak with their employer to understand their rights and any company-specific provisions regarding time off for medical needs.

However, employers may offer flexibility, but it is not mandated by law unless explicitly stated in the employee's contract. Many employers will allow time off if an employee cannot rearrange their appointment. The time off might be unpaid.

Source: www.acas.org.uk/time-off-for-medical-appointments

QUESTION 46

You are asked to see a welder who is concerned about his risk of cancer from welding fumes after seeing an alert on TikTok.

What is the commonest type of cancer associated with welding fumes?

The answer is: e) Lung cancer

Welding is a common occupational activity in the UK and gives rise to a complex mixture of readily respirable fumes. The composition of the fume is determined by the welding process, by the metals (and any coating they may have) that are being fused, and by the nature of any filler material and shielding gas. Some welding fumes, such as those from stainless steel welding, contain recognised lung carcinogens (e.g. hexavalent chromium).

The International Agency for Research on Cancer (IARC) classifies both welding fumes and ultraviolet (UV) radiation from welding as Group 1 carcinogens, the agency's designation for agents that carry sufficient evidence of carcinogenicity in humans. According to the monograph, welding fumes cause lung cancer, and positive associations have been observed with kidney cancer. UV radiation from welding can cause ocular melanoma.

For all other cancers, studies considered by IARC presented inadequate evidence for the carcinogenicity of welding fumes.

Source: www.hse.gov.uk/welding/health-risks-welding.htm

QUESTION 47

You are reviewing a pre-placement health questionnaire for an individual applying to work as a baker. The individual has a history of atopy.

What is the most appropriate next action you should take?

The answer is: a) Fit for work

Atopy is common (30% of the population); it is not usually appropriate to screen out atopics from exposure to sensitising agents at pre-employment.

Source: Sadhra, S., Bray, A.J. and Boorman, S. (eds) (2022) *Oxford Handbook of Occupational Health*, third edition

QUESTION 48

You are implementing a screening programme for Covid-19 in a workplace. The Covid-19 test has a sensitivity of 90% and a specificity of 98%. You need to explain these statistics to the employer.
Which one of the following best explains the sensitivity of the Covid-19 test to the employer?

The answer is: a) 90% of people with a Covid-19 infection will test positive on the test

Sensitivity refers to the percentage of true positives (people who have the disease) who are correctly identified by the test. In this case, 90% of individuals with Covid-19 will test positive, which is why option a) is correct.

Specificity refers to the percentage of true negatives (people who do not have the disease) who are correctly identified. While specificity is important, it is not directly relevant to the question asked in this case.

Source: https://blogs.imperial.ac.uk/medical-centre/2023/10/10/making-sense-of-sensitivity-specificity-and-predictive-value-a-guide-for-patients-clinicians-and-policymakers

QUESTION 49

You are asked to help set up the first aid provisions in a charity shop employing twenty people.

You are asked to provide an opinion on the type of training needed for first aiders.

Which is the most likely training needed under the First Aid Regulations?

The answer is: b) Emergency first aid at work

This framework helps organisations determine the appropriate level of first aid coverage based on the number of employees and the risk level of the workplace under the First Aid Regulations 1981.

- **Degree of hazard**:
    - *Low-hazard workplaces* (e.g. offices, shops, libraries):
        - fewer than 25 employees: at least 1 appointed person
        - 25–50 employees: at least 1 EFAW (Emergency First Aid at Work) trained first aider
        - more than 50 employees: at least 1 FAW (First Aid at Work) trained first aider per 100 employees (or part thereof).
    - *higher hazard workplaces* (e.g. light engineering, food processing, construction):
        - fewer than 5 employees: at least 1 appointed person
        - 5–50 employees: at least 1 EFAW or FAW trained first aider, depending on the type of injuries that may occur
        - more than 50 employees: at least 1 FAW trained first aider per 50 employees (or part thereof).
- **Additional considerations**:
    - Factors affecting first aid provisions include the presence of inexperienced workers, employees with disabilities, those working remotely or alone, and the layout or location of the workplace.

Source: www.hse.gov.uk/pubns/priced/l74.pdf

QUESTION 50

A construction worker complains of symptoms suggestive of carpal tunnel syndrome (CTS) and on examination shows symptoms suggestive of sensorineural hand arm vibration syndrome (HAVS).

Answers to Mock exam 3

What is the most appropriate next step?

The answer is: c) Refer for further assessment of CTS

When a worker presents with both CTS and symptoms indicative of sensorineural HAVS, the immediate priority is to address and treat the CTS first. The presence of CTS can affect the evaluation and grading of HAVS. Therefore, referring the worker for a comprehensive assessment and treatment of CTS is crucial before proceeding to evaluate the severity of HAVS. Once CTS is managed, the severity of HAVS can be more accurately assessed.

Source: www.som.org.uk/sites/som.org.uk/files/Carpal_tunnel_syndrome_and_work_with_hand-held_vibrating_tools_Jan2022.pdf

QUESTION 51

A 58-year-old office worker has been on extended medical leave due to a chronic illness. The company has referred you to consider the employee for ill-health retirement under the company's pension scheme.

Which one of the following actions should the medical practitioner prioritise when assessing the employee's eligibility for an early retirement pension?

The answer is: d) Review the company pension scheme eligibility criteria

The medical practitioner must begin by thoroughly reviewing the company pension scheme's eligibility criteria to understand the specific requirements and conditions for ill-health retirement. This step ensures that the assessment is consistent with the pension scheme's rules. It is essential to review these criteria before conducting any medical assessments or forming an opinion based on the employee's health status or other information.

Source: Hobson, J. and Smedley, J. (eds) (2019) *Fitness for Work: the medical aspects*, 6th edition. Oxford University Press

QUESTION 52

A manufacturing company conducts routine noise surveillance for its employees to monitor and protect their hearing health. The OH team is reviewing various methods and tests used in their programme.

Which one of the following is NOT part of routine noise surveillance?

The answer is: a) Otoacoustic emission (OAE) tests

OAE testing is specialised and used for early detection of hearing damage, particularly in infants, and is not typically part of routine noise surveillance in occupational settings.

Questionnaires are used to gather information on symptoms or changes in hearing, making them a common part of routine noise surveillance.

Pure tone audiometry is a fundamental part of routine noise surveillance, used to measure hearing thresholds and assess any hearing loss.

Otoscopic examination checks the ear canal and eardrum for physical issues, and is a standard part of routine noise surveillance before conducting audiometric tests.

Health promotion involves educating employees about hearing protection and noise exposure, which is an integral component of a noise surveillance programme.

Source: www.hse.gov.uk/pubns/priced/l108.pdf

QUESTION 53

While conducting a training session for new employees on workplace health and safety measures, you describe the hierarchy of control.

Which of the following controls is considered the control of last resort?

The answer is: c) Personal protective equipment (PPE)

PPE is considered a last resort because it addresses exposure at an individual level rather than controlling the hazard at its source, which would benefit all in the area.

Additionally, PPE's effectiveness can vary, and assessing the actual protection level can be challenging.

PPE may also restrict movement and visibility, which could interfere with work tasks.

Lastly, for PPE to provide effective protection, it must be correctly chosen, fitted, used and maintained.

Source: Sadhra, S., Bray, A.J. and Boorman, S. (eds) (2022) *Oxford Handbook of Occupational Health*, third edition

QUESTION 54

A company that works with ionising radiation is conducting baseline medical surveillance to assess the fitness of its employees for their intended work.

Which of the following factors is most relevant to assess in detail when undertaking baseline health surveillance for work with ionising radiation (IR)?

The answer is: d) Whether the employee has a history of previous significant medical exposure to ionising radiation

The main purpose of this consultation is to establish the fitness of the individual to work with ionising radiation.

A full medical history should be obtained at this consultation.

Key aspects related to work involving IR, and which should therefore be assessed in this consultation, include a history of:
- chronic skin disease
- chronic pulmonary disease
- psychiatric illness or personality disorder
- blood disorders
- inherited predisposition to malignancy
- medical exposure to IR
- treatment with cytotoxic drugs
- diagnostic and therapeutic exposures to IR
- occupational exposures to IR or other carcinogens (e.g. asbestos).

Other relevant factors to be considered at this consultation include the employee's ability to wear the required PPE (including RPE) necessary for protection against ionising radiation.

On this basis, neurological and cardiovascular disease and manual dexterity are not as relevant.

QUESTION 55

You are working with a large law firm to help them tender for a new OH provider. You are discussing the importance of accreditation and quality standards in OH services during a team meeting when an HR colleague asks about a specific accreditation standard that is widely recognised in the UK, SEQOHS.

What does SEQOHS stand for?

The answer is: c) Safe Effective Quality Occupational Health Service

The Safe Effective Quality Occupational Health Service (SEQOHS) is a recognised voluntary accreditation scheme that sets the standard for OH services in the UK. SEQOHS ensures that OH providers meet robust criteria for safety, quality and effectiveness. The accreditation is applicable to both public and private sector providers, helping to foster trust and continuous improvement in OH practices.

Providers pursuing SEQOHS accreditation undergo an independent assessment based on well-defined standards, including clinical governance, information security and staff competency. This process drives improvement and ensures services deliver high-quality support to employees and employers alike. Accreditation is valid for 5 years, subject to annual review, and providers benefit from external validation, enhanced reputation, and opportunities to showcase best practice.

Source: www.fom.ac.uk/media-events/publications/seqohs-publications

QUESTION 56

As part of his pre-placement health screening of health workers you see a locum consultant who has come to the UK in the last year from a low-TB incidence country.

What is the most appropriate first step in his assessment to ensure he does not have tuberculosis (TB)?

The answer is: c) Enquire about a personal or family history of TB

Clinical students, agency, locum staff and contract ancillary workers with patient or clinical material contact should undergo TB screening at the same standards as permanent NHS employees.

Taking a history is the next step before any investigations.

All employees new to the NHS are required to undergo TB screening or provide documentation of screening conducted within the past 12 months before starting work with patients or clinical specimens.

Health checks for new NHS employees who will have patient or clinical material contact should include:
- assessment of personal or family history of TB
- inquiry into symptoms and signs, potentially through a questionnaire
- verification of tuberculin skin testing (or interferon-gamma testing) and/or BCG scar check by an OH professional, not solely relying on the applicant's assessment
- tuberculin skin test (or interferon-gamma test) result within the last 5 years, if available.

Employees without clear evidence of prior BCG vaccination should undergo a Mantoux tuberculin skin test (or interferon-gamma test).

Source: https://assets.publishing.service.gov.uk/media/5a7ed8d5e5274a2e87db2479/health_clearance_tuberculosis_hepatitis_hiv.pdf

QUESTION 57

You are an OH specialist reviewing a study conducted to investigate the potential link between exposure to a hazardous chemical in the workplace and the development of a specific type of cancer. The study involved identifying workers who have already developed the cancer and a comparison group of workers who do not have the cancer. The investigators then looked back at their exposure histories to determine if there was a higher prevalence of exposure to the hazardous chemical among those who developed the cancer.

What type of study design best describes the method used in this investigation?

The answer is: d) Case–control study

A case–control study is designed to compare individuals with a specific condition (cases) to those without the condition (controls) and then look back retrospectively to assess their exposure to potential risk factors. In this case, the study design fits the description of a case–control study, as it involved comparing the exposure histories of workers who developed cancer with those who did not.

Source: www.cebm.ox.ac.uk/resources/ebm-tools/study-designs

QUESTION 58

A factory employs workers exposed to various hazardous substances, including lead and asbestos. Management is reviewing regulatory requirements for medical surveillance to ensure compliance.

Under which of the following regulations might medical surveillance by an appointed doctor be required?

The answer is: b) Control of Asbestos Regulations 2012

An appointed doctor is a registered medical practitioner appointed by the HSE to undertake statutory medical surveillance. The HSE is responsible for the following regulations where medical surveillance conducted by an appointed doctor may be required:
- Ionising Radiations Regulations 2017
- Control of Lead at Work Regulations 2002
- Control of Asbestos Regulations 2012
- Control of Substances Hazardous to Health Regulations 2002 (as amended)
- Work in Compressed Air Regulations 1996

Source: www.hse.gov.uk/doctors/information.htm

QUESTION 59

You are assessing a 48-year-old lorry driver for a renewal of his licence with a diagnosis of angina. Whilst in the waiting room you notice that he needs to use his GTN spray.

In the consultation room you inform him that you cannot renew his licence as he has ongoing chest pain, and that he needs to inform the DVLA. He refuses to accept this and tells you that he needs to have his licence renewed or he will lose his job.

What is the most appropriate next step?

The answer is: b) Arrange a second opinion on his fitness to drive

DVLA guidance states that you should do the following:

Inform the patient:
- Clearly explain to the patient how their medical condition or ongoing treatment affects their ability to drive safely.

- Tell them that they have a legal duty to notify the Driver and Vehicle Licensing Agency (DVLA) of any condition that affects their driving ability. Ensure they understand the seriousness of this responsibility.

Warn the patient:
- Advise the patient that if they continue to drive while unfit, you might have to disclose relevant medical information to the DVLA.
- Emphasise that this information will be shared confidentially and only with the appropriate authorities to ensure road safety.

Document advice:
- Medical record notation: make detailed notes in the patient's medical record about the advice given regarding their fitness to drive. This should include the date, the specifics of the advice, and the patient's response or any actions they plan to take.

Dispute of diagnosis:
- If the patient disputes the diagnosis or its impact on their driving, suggest that they seek a second opinion from another healthcare professional.
- Advise the patient to refrain from driving until the second opinion is obtained.
- With the patient's agreement, discuss your concerns about their fitness to drive with their relatives, friends or carers to ensure a support system is aware and can help manage the situation.

Continuing to drive unfit:
- Make every reasonable effort to persuade the patient to stop driving if you believe they are unfit.
- If the patient continues to drive against your advice, assess whether their refusal to stop driving poses a significant risk of death or serious harm to themselves or others.
- Confidential reporting: if such a risk is present, promptly contact the DVLA or DVA and provide the necessary medical information confidentially to their medical adviser.

Notify before disclosure:
- Before contacting the DVLA, try to inform the patient about your intention to disclose their medical information.
- Listen to any objections the patient may have and weigh their reasons carefully.

- After deciding to contact the DVLA, inform the patient in writing that the disclosure has been made.
- Record all these actions and the rationale in the patient's medical record to maintain a clear and traceable history of your decision-making process and communication with the patient.

Sources:
- www.gov.uk/guidance/cardiovascular-disorders-assessing-fitness-to-drive
- www.gmc-uk.org/professional-standards/the-professional-standards/confidentiality---patients-fitness-to-drive-and-reporting-concerns-to-the-dvla-or-dva/patients-fitness-to-drive-and-reporting-concerns-to-the-dvla-or-dva

QUESTION 60

You are an OH professional conducting a risk assessment for a 35-year-old factory worker with managerial duties who has recently been diagnosed with epilepsy. The worker's seizures are currently not well-controlled, and you need to determine the appropriate work restrictions to ensure their safety.

Which of the following work activities is most appropriate to restrict for an employee with poorly-controlled epilepsy?

The answer is: d) Driving a forklift in a warehouse environment

Driving a forklift poses a significant risk for someone with epilepsy if seizures are not well-controlled. Operating motorised machinery is explicitly restricted due to the high risk of accidents that could result from a seizure occurring while the vehicle is in motion.

Clerical work at a desk with occasional computer use is generally safe for individuals with epilepsy, as it does not involve any significant risks related to the typical triggers or hazards associated with seizures.

Operating a hand-held power tool with an automatic shut-off feature: the use of any hand-held powered tool should be carefully considered for someone with epilepsy, especially if the tool can cause injury if left in the 'on' position during a seizure. However, the automatic shut-off feature makes it less hazardous.

Supervising other workers while standing on the ground floor: supervisory roles that do not involve physical hazards such as heights, water or machinery are typically safe for individuals with epilepsy, assuming they are in a safe environment.

Performing routine inventory checks in a storage room might be safe, depending on the environment and specific risks present (such as heights, unguarded machinery or water), but generally, inventory checks in a controlled environment without specific hazards would not require restriction.

For individuals with epilepsy, particularly if their condition is not well-controlled, restrictions should focus on activities that involve significant safety risks, such as driving, operating machinery, working at heights or near water or fire, and using hand-held tools that could cause injury during a seizure.

Source: Hobson, J. and Smedley, J. (eds) (2019) *Fitness for Work: the medical aspects*, 6th edition. Oxford University Press

QUESTION 61

As the senior OHP, you are approached by a new medical administrator in your department who is archiving old records. She seeks clarification on how long the clinical records of employees should be retained for. Her main concern is ensuring compliance with the specific regulatory requirements governing OH records.

For how long should these records be retained?

The answer is: c) Either until 6 years after retirement or until they reach 75 years of age, whichever is sooner

Under GDPR, personal data, including OH records, must be retained only for as long as necessary for their processing purposes. Guidance from the Information Governance Alliance / Department of Health suggests retaining OH records for the duration of the person's employment plus 6 years or until their 75th birthday, whichever is sooner.

In contrast, records of statutory health surveillance under specific regulations (e.g. COSHH, Control of Vibration, Control of Noise, Control of Lead, Control of Asbestos, and Ionising Radiations Regulations) require employers to maintain basic health records for 40 years (30 years for ionising radiations). The detailed clinical records with the results of the tests and other clinical information should be kept separate in the confidential OH record and not disclosed without consent. The health record should be kept for 40 years (30 years in the case of ionising radiations) but the clinical records do not need to be retained for as long as that unless there is, exceptionally, a special reason for doing so. Detailed clinical records from these surveillance activities, however, need not be retained for as long unless specific reasons warrant their extended retention.

Source: www.fom.ac.uk/media-events/news/guidance/guidance-on-the-general-data-protection-regulation

QUESTION 62

An office worker is about to undergo total hip replacement surgery and has been proactively referred for advice so that the team can plan for her absence.

According to guidance on returning to work after hip replacement surgery, which of the following is the most appropriate advice for an uncomplicated recovery?

The answer is: b) They can typically return to work within 4–6 weeks if their job involves mostly sedentary activities and they follow their surgeon's advice

Every person recovers differently and has different needs. In most cases it's usually safe to return to light work or an office-based job within 6 weeks of the operation.

Source: Sadhra, S., Bray, A.J. and Boorman, S. (eds) (2022) *Oxford Handbook of Occupational Health*, third edition

QUESTION 63

A trainee nurse has sustained a high-risk needlestick injury. Management is seeking advice on any work restrictions that should be imposed during the follow-up testing period.

What is the best advice you should give management regarding restrictions on the trainee nurse during their follow-up tests?

The answer is: c) They can continue to work without restrictions during the follow-up period

Recipients of high-risk needlestick injuries should not be restricted from work (or EPPs) during follow-up.

Source: Sadhra, S., Bray, A.J. and Boorman, S. (eds) (2022) *Oxford Handbook of Occupational Health*, third edition

QUESTION 64

You are giving a lecture about the risks of ultraviolet (UV) radiation.

In which one of the following occupations is there a statistically significant increased risk of ocular melanoma?

The answer is: c) Welders

Increased risks have been reported in several occupational groups with high exposures to UV radiation. These include construction workers, sailors and fishermen, agricultural workers, airline pilots and those exposed to electromagnetic radiation. Other occupations for which an increased risk has been suggested include chemists, healthcare workers, laundry workers and service workers. For none of these occupations, however, is the evidence both strong and consistent.

In contrast, there is a more coherent body of evidence in relation to two other occupational activities: welding and cooking.

Welders, especially those involved in arc welding, have the most robust evidence linking their occupational exposures to an increased risk of ocular melanoma. This increased risk is attributed to both high levels of UV radiation and exposure to carcinogenic substances such as hexavalent chromium and thorium oxide, as confirmed by the International Agency for Research on Cancer (IARC) in 2012.

Source: https://assets.publishing.service.gov.uk/media/5a7eadc840f0b62305b82796/ocular-melanoma-and-occupation-iiac-pp-33.pdf

QUESTION 65

You are teaching a group of medical students about the Equality Act 2010 and its role in protecting individuals from discrimination in the workplace and other settings.

Which one of the following is a protected characteristic under the Equality Act 2010?

The answer is: a) Gender reassignment

The Equality Act 2010 lists nine protected characteristics, including gender reassignment, to prevent discrimination based on various aspects of a person's identity. These characteristics are: age, disability, gender reassignment, marriage and civil partnership, pregnancy and maternity, race, religion or belief, sex, and sexual orientation.

Source: www.acas.org.uk/discrimination-and-the-law

QUESTION 66

You are evaluating the performance of a new diagnostic test for a workplace health surveillance programme. In a population of 1000 individuals, 100 are confirmed to have the disease based on a gold standard test. The new diagnostic test correctly identifies 80 individuals with the disease.

What is the sensitivity of the diagnostic test?

The answer is: d) 80%

Sensitivity measures the ability of a test to correctly identify those with the disease. It is calculated as:

Sensitivity = true positives / (true positives + false negatives)

For this test:
- True positives (TP): 80
- False negatives (FN): 20 (individuals with the disease who were missed by the test).

Sensitivity = 80 / (80 + 20)

Thus, the sensitivity of the test is 80%.

Source: https://blogs.imperial.ac.uk/medical-centre/2023/10/10/making-sense-of-sensitivity-specificity-and-predictive-value-a-guide-for-patients-clinicians-and-policymakers

QUESTION 67

You are reviewing the spirometry results of a 55-year-old employee who presents for health surveillance with a history of chronic cough and shortness of breath.

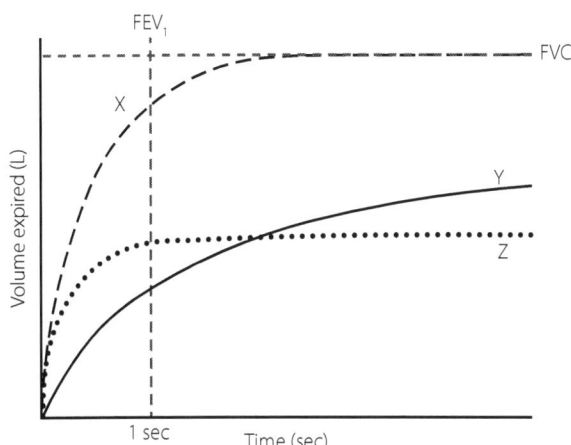

The spirometry is represented by line Y on the graph.

What is the most likely pathology?

The answer is: e) Obstructive disease

The pattern shown by line Y in the spirometry graph represents obstructive disease. This condition is characterised by a significant reduction in FEV_1, while forced vital capacity (FVC) may be relatively preserved. As a result, the FEV_1/FVC ratio is reduced, which is typical of conditions such as chronic obstructive pulmonary disease (COPD) or asthma. This contrasts with restrictive disease, where both FEV_1 and FVC are reduced, but the FEV_1/FVC ratio is typically normal or increased. X is normal spirometry and Z is a restrictive pattern.

QUESTION 68

You are conducting a training session on occupational toxicology for a group of new employees at a chemical manufacturing plant. During the session, you explain that understanding toxicokinetics is essential for assessing the potential health effects of chemical exposures.

What are the four components of toxicokinetics?

The answer is: a) Absorption, Distribution, Metabolism, Excretion

The four processes of absorption, distribution, metabolism and excretion are the primary components of toxicokinetics. They determine the concentration of a substance at target sites in the body, influencing the toxicity level.

QUESTION 69

A junior health and safety officer reviewing workplace procedures for managing exposure to hazardous substances asks you where they can find the official workplace exposure limits (WELs) to ensure compliance with current regulations.

What is the most appropriate answer?

The answer is: c) EH40

The EH40 is the official source for WELs in the UK. It is published by the Health and Safety Executive (HSE). It helps ensure that employers and workers can effectively manage exposure to hazardous substances.

Source: www.hse.gov.uk/pubns/priced/eh40.pdf

QUESTION 70

As part of your research project on occupational cancers in the UK, you are reviewing previous research on the industry with the highest incidence of occupational cancer cases.

Based on current evidence, which UK industry is known to have the highest burden of occupational cancers?

The answer is: b) Construction

The construction industry has the largest burden of occupational cancers amongst the industrial sectors. Over 40% of the occupational cancer deaths and cancer registrations were from the industry. Most cancers in construction were lung cancers caused by exposure to asbestos and silica. A significant number of lung (and other) cancers are also linked to diesel engine exhaust emissions.

Source: www.hse.gov.uk/construction/healthrisks/cancer-and-construction/key-points.htm

Answers to Mock exam 3

QUESTION 71

An employer is developing a strategy to manage dust exposure in the workplace and needs to understand the order of priority for implementing control measures to effectively reduce exposure to dust.

In managing dust exposure, which one of the following control measures should be prioritised?

The answer is: d) Enclose the process so that dust does not escape

Control measures usually involve a combination of equipment and ways of working to reduce exposure. The right combination is crucial. No measures, however practical, can work unless they are used properly.

In order of priority the right combination of control measures could include:
1. Eliminate the use of a harmful product or substance and use a safer one.
2. Use a safer form of the product, e.g. paste rather than powder.
3. Change the process to emit less of the substance.
4. Enclose the process so that dust does not escape.
5. Extract dust emissions near the source.
6. Minimise the number of workers that are at risk.
7. Apply suitable administrative controls, such as reducing the length of time that workers are exposed to dust.
8. Provide personal protective equipment (PPE) such as gloves, coveralls and a respirator. PPE must fit the wearer. The provision of PPE, if required, should be in addition to the measures above, not instead of.

Source: www.hse.gov.uk/dust/assets/docs/eh44.pdf

QUESTION 72

You are assisting a large manufacturing company in updating its food handler policy. Management is looking for a precise definition of a 'food handler' to ensure the policy is clear and comprehensive.

What is the best definition of a 'food handler'?

The answer is: b) A person who manufactures, prepares or transports food and may come into direct contact with food or with machines handling unwrapped food

A 'food handler' is defined as someone involved in the manufacturing, preparation or transportation of food who may either directly touch the food itself or interact with machinery that handles unwrapped food. This definition includes engineers, cleaners and those visiting the premises. The definition also includes those preparing or serving food in canteens and shops.

Source: Sadhra, S., Bray, A.J. and Boorman, S. (eds) (2022) *Oxford Handbook of Occupational Health*, third edition

QUESTION 73

You are the OHP seeing an 18-year-old gardener who has exceeded her sickness absence threshold due to frequent absences from work. She has recently developed symptoms of seasonal allergic rhinitis during the spring and summer seasons. Her symptoms include frequent sneezing, itchy and watery eyes, and nasal congestion, which pose significant challenges for her while working outdoors in gardens with high pollen levels. Despite starting antihistamines recently, she has not experienced relief from her symptoms. She does not have any other medical conditions.

What is the most suitable advice to include in your report concerning the Equality Act 2010?

The answer is: d) Seasonal allergic rhinitis is not covered as a disability under the Equality Act 2010, except where it aggravates the effects of another condition

Seasonal allergic rhinitis, commonly known as hay fever, is generally excluded from being considered a disability under the Equality Act 2010. This means that individuals who experience hay fever symptoms during certain seasons do not qualify for legal protections against discrimination based solely on this condition. However, if hay fever exacerbates the effects of another underlying condition that meets the criteria for disability under the Act (such as asthma or chronic sinusitis), then the effects of hay fever may be taken into consideration.

Other exclusions from the definition of disability as defined by the Equality Act 2010:
- addiction to, or dependency on, alcohol, nicotine, or any other substance (other than in consequence of the substance being medically prescribed)
- tendency to set fires
- tendency to steal

- tendency to physical or sexual abuse of other persons
- exhibitionism
- voyeurism.

Source: www.gov.uk/government/publications/equality-act-guidance/disability-equality-act-2010-guidance-on-matters-to-be-taken-into-account-in-determining-questions-relating-to-the-definition-of-disability-html

QUESTION 74

During a consultation, an employee undergoing her third round of *in vitro* fertilisation (IVF) treatment expresses frustration because her managers are not allowing her paid time off to attend IVF-related medical appointments. She mentions that this is causing conflict in the team, as pregnant employees are being given paid time off for antenatal appointments. The employee has been referred to you for work-related stress due to this situation.

What is the most appropriate response regarding the employee's rights to time off for IVF treatment?

The answer is: b) There is no legal right to paid time off for IVF treatment, but the employer should be encouraged to treat this the same as any other medical appointment or sickness absence

While there is no specific legal right for employees to receive paid time off for IVF treatment or related sickness, Acas (the Advisory, Conciliation and Arbitration Service) advises that employers are encouraged to treat such medical appointments and any related sickness absence the same as they would any other medical issue. This includes allowing reasonable time off for appointments and treating any related sickness absence fairly.

This approach helps to support employees undergoing IVF while maintaining a fair and consistent policy for all types of medical leave within the workplace.

Source: www.acas.org.uk/your-maternity-leave-pay-and-other-rights/having-ivf-treatment

QUESTION 75

During a training session for health and safety officers, you explain that certain exposures in the workplace contribute more significantly to cancer-related deaths than others. You highlight that, according to recent data, one substance is responsible for the highest number of occupational cancer deaths in the UK.

Which one of the following is the leading cause of occupational cancer deaths in Great Britain?

The answer is: e) Asbestos

Asbestos exposure is the leading cause of occupational cancer deaths in Great Britain, primarily due to its strong association with lung cancer and mesothelioma.

The following graph from the HSE (2024) shows the estimated occupational cancer deaths by cause in Great Britain, highlighting that past asbestos exposure remains the leading cause of deaths from occupational cancer in Great Britain. Other significant contributors include exposure to silica, solar radiation, mineral oils and shift work. The construction industry is particularly affected, with an estimated 3500 cancer deaths in 2005 and 5500 cancer registrations in 2004.

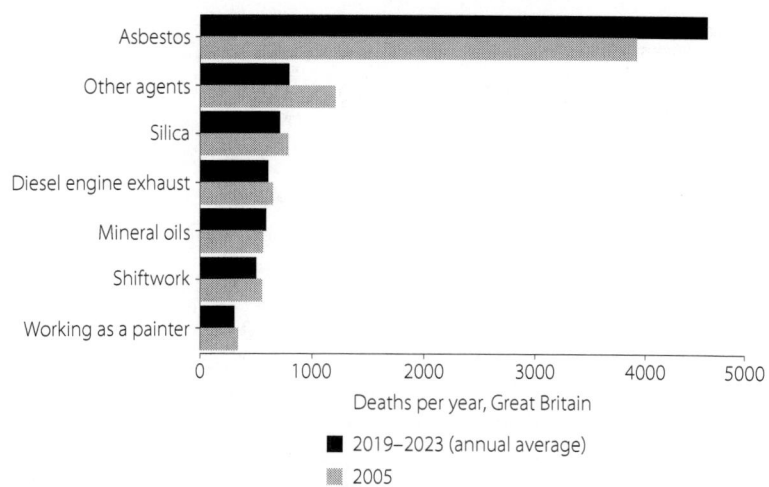

Public sector information published by the Health and Safety Executive and licensed under the Open Government Licence.

Source: www.hse.gov.uk/statistics/assets/docs/cancer.pdf

QUESTION 76

You are an OHP undertaking an assessment of a 30-year-old industrial radiographer who has recently notified her employer that she is pregnant.

What is the most appropriate action the employer should take?

The answer is: c) Make sure that the pregnant employee's work conditions are adjusted to ensure the foetal dose is unlikely to exceed 1 mSv during the remainder of the pregnancy

Ionising Radiations Regulations 2017 concerning pregnant employees working with ionising radiation require that the employer adjust work conditions to ensure that the equivalent dose to the foetus is ALARP and remains below 1 mSv during the remainder of the pregnancy. This is to minimise the risk of harm to the developing foetus.

Source: www.hse.gov.uk/pubns/books/l121.htm

QUESTION 77

A worker has been diagnosed with a condition that may be reportable.

Which one of the following conditions is not classified as a reportable occupational disease under RIDDOR?

The answer is: d) Noise-induced hearing loss

The Reporting of Injuries, Diseases, and Dangerous Occurrences Regulations (RIDDOR) require employers and self-employed individuals to report certain occupational diseases if these are linked to specified workplace hazards. The diseases must be confirmed by a doctor and are reportable only if they result from work-related exposures.

Reportable diseases:

Carpal tunnel syndrome: reportable if caused by regular use of hand-held power tools involving repetitive blows or vibrations, not from typing or similar repetitive movements.

Cramp of the hand or forearm: reportable if chronic and caused by prolonged repetitive movements.

Occupational dermatitis: reportable if caused by significant exposure to skin irritants or sensitisers, such as chemicals in various industries.

Hand arm vibration syndrome: reportable if caused by regular exposure to vibrating tools or machines.

Occupational asthma: reportable if caused by significant exposure to known respiratory sensitisers.

Tendonitis or tenosynovitis: reportable if it affects the hand or forearm and results from frequent, repetitive movements or physically demanding work.

Diseases caused by exposure to carcinogens, mutagens or biological agents must also be reported.

Conditions linked to non-work-related exposures or not involving the specified workplace hazards are not reportable.

Source: www.hse.gov.uk/riddor/occupational-diseases.htm

QUESTION 78

You are seeing a 35-year-old factory worker with well-controlled insulin-dependent diabetes. He has been referred for advice on whether he can safely work rotating shifts, and he is eager to start as soon as possible.

What is the most appropriate advice for you to provide regarding his suitability for working on rotating shifts?

The answer is: c) He can work rotating shifts but may need to make adjustments to his meal schedule and glucose monitoring

For individuals with well-controlled insulin-dependent diabetes, modern insulin regimens allow for flexibility, making rotating shifts feasible.

Sources:
- www.cdc.gov/diabetes/articles/diabetes-shift-work.html
- Sadhra, S., Bray, A.J. and Boorman, S. (eds) (2022) *Oxford Handbook of Occupational Health*, third edition

QUESTION 79

A 32-year-old office worker, who is 28 weeks pregnant, has been referred to you for advice on workplace adjustments. She has recently been started on insulin for gestational diabetes. She is under the care of both an obstetrician and an endocrinologist, and so far she has not experienced any disabling hypoglycaemic events, and is not expected to experience any. She is concerned about how her condition and insulin treatment might affect her ability to drive safely on her 20-minute commute to work.

What is the most appropriate advice regarding her driving while being treated with insulin?

The answer is: b) She may continue driving and does not need to notify the DVLA

For temporary insulin treatment, including for the treatment of gestational diabetes:

Group 1 drivers (cars and motorcycles):
- May drive without notifying the DVLA if:
    - they are under medical supervision
    - they are not considered at risk of disabling hypoglycaemia by their clinician
- Must notify the DVLA if:
    - disabling hypoglycaemia occurs
    - treatment continues for more than 3 months, or for gestational diabetes, if it continues for more than 3 months after delivery.

Group 2 drivers (buses and lorries):
- Must notify the DVLA and meet the above standards.

Source: www.gov.uk/diabetes-driving

QUESTION 80

You are reviewing the pre-placement questionnaire of a nurse who was born and raised in the UK and has applied for a role at the local hospital. The nurse has indicated that she had chickenpox at the age of 5.

What is the most appropriate next step?

The answer is: d) No further action needed, she can be cleared to work

According to the guidelines referenced below, for healthcare workers (HCWs) who were born and raised in temperate climates, such as the UK, a positive history of chickenpox or shingles is generally considered sufficient evidence of immunity to VZV. Since the nurse has confirmed that she had chickenpox at the age of 5 and was born and brought up in the UK, no further serological testing is required, and she can be cleared to work.

Arranging an appointment to clarify the history of chickenpox is unnecessary because the nurse has already provided a clear positive history of chickenpox, which is considered sufficient evidence of immunity.

Although serological testing is recommended for HCWs from tropical or subtropical climates or those with an uncertain history, it is not needed in this case because the nurse's positive history of chickenpox is accepted as proof of immunity.

Source: www.nhshealthatwork.co.uk/images/library/files/Clinical%20excellence/Varicella_zoster_guidelines_web_navigable.pdf

Excel in your Occupational Health exams with confidence!

Dr Clare Fernandes, Co-Director of **The Occupational Health Academy**, invites you to enhance your preparation with two expertly crafted courses. Created by **Dr Fernandes** and **Dr Chowdhury**, these sessions are packed with **practical advice, real-world examples and expert insights**. Past attendees have consistently achieved **top scores**, and glowing reviews speak for themselves.

DOccMed Portfolio Morning

Struggling with your **FOM portfolio**? This session is your ultimate guide to success, offering:

- ☑ **Step-by-step guidance** for selecting the right workplace and clinical case.
- ☑ Tips to **structure your portfolio** – concise, impactful and exam-ready.
- ☑ Insights into how your portfolio prepares you for the **Mock Viva** – making the process smoother.
- ☑ Examples of **high-scoring portfolios** to inspire and guide your own work.
- ☑ An engaging **Q&A session** to address all your portfolio concerns.

DOccMed MCQ Weekend

Feeling overwhelmed by the vast syllabus or unsure about key occupational health concepts? This popular course covers:

- ☑ Core principles in **OH Ethics and Law, Occupational Hygiene** and **Occupational Medicine**.
- ☑ Expert **exam tips** and insights on **past topics** to boost your preparation.
- ☑ High-yield content designed to **save time** while improving focus.
- ☑ Strategies to confidently tackle even the **toughest MCQs**.
- ☑ **Exclusive offer for SOM members**
- ☑ **Save 20% on course fees!** Log in to your SOM account before registering to access the discount, or email membership@som.org.uk for assistance.

Don't wait—register today and take the first step toward portfolio and exam success!

For further course details and reviews, see:
https://occupationalhealthacademy.co.uk

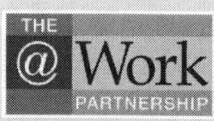

Take your OH career further with The At Work Partnership

High quality training, qualifications & information for OH professionals

Specialists in providing expert information to OH professionals, we run a number of high quality, good value conferences as well as specialist professional development courses to help you progress in your occupational health career. We also publish the bi-monthly journal Occupational Health [at Work].

OH Conferences & events

Our courses on occupational health and disability issues are designed to help OH practitioners to continuously develop and enhance their practice.

Courses include:
OH Report Writing, Hand-Arm Vibration Syndrome courses, OH consultations as well as Certificates in Managing OH services, OH Law, OH Case Management and Managing Mental Health at Work.

Occupational Health [at Work] journal

Designed to make your working life easier, the Occupational Health [at Work] journal provides the OH management, legal and medical information you need!

Recent journal articles have covered: *Consent to release OH reports, artificial intelligence, dyslexia and work, returning to work after cancer, mental health, suicide ideation, disability discrimination & much more...*

Contact us or visit our site for information on courses & journal subscriptions

 www.atworkpartnership.co.uk info@atworkpartnership.co.uk

Diploma in Occupational Medicine
Ten Day Virtual Training Course

Are you looking to become a specialist in Occupational Health?

The RSPH is approved by the Faculty of Occupational Medicine (FOM) to run the FOM course to prepare candidates for the Diploma in Occupational Medicine's written examination and the oral examination based on a portfolio. This is a ten day intensive course available to candidates wishing to sit the exam for the Diploma in Occupational Medicine professional qualification.

AIMS
The FOM Diploma has been designed for registered practitioners. It demonstrates that the holder has achieved a competence appropriate to a generalist working in occupational health. This course is the foundation level qualification required for occupational medicine.

Course content and objectives
- Epidemiology
- Occupational lung
- Occupational skin disease
- Disability assessment
- Musculoskeletal disorders
- Toxicology
- Biological monitoring
- Occupational mental health disorders
- The examination
- Industrial relations
- Occupational health law
- Ethics

By the end of the course, participants should:
- be competent to seek and apply special information and techniques in Occupational medicine;
- be conversant with current thinking on the application of appropriate legislation;
- satisfy all the requirements of the Faculty's Diploma Core Syllabus.

TUTORS
Our Course Director Dr Shriti Pattani leads a distinguished group of tutors and speakers who cover a wide range of occupational medicine/health specialties. Speakers include senior occupational medical officers with experience in organisations such as the Health & Safety Executive, the Foreign & Commonwealth Office and past FOM examiners; along with consultants in occupational medicine, health and safety, toxicology and epidemiology, specialists in occupational health and hygiene.
You will also have several sessions by representatives of the Faculty who discuss the whole qualification; a mock exam is given at the end of the course and advice is given on how to write the portfolio for the oral examination.

FEE AND BOOKING
Please visit the RSPH website www.rsph.org.uk/events

Registered Charity number 1125949

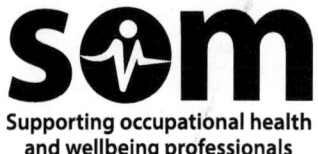

Supporting occupational health and wellbeing professionals

Join as a member today

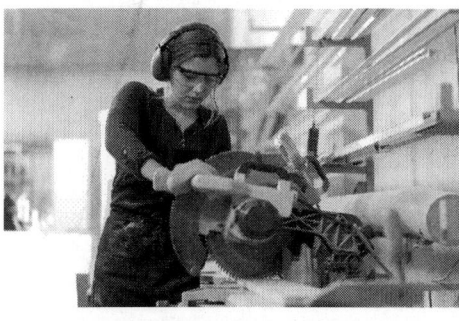
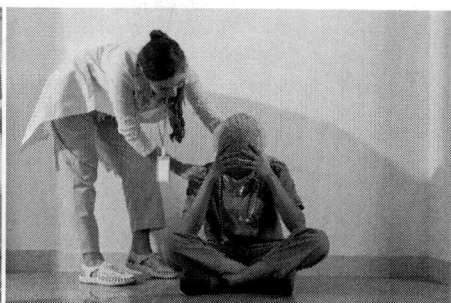

Are you a healthcare professional working in occupational health and medicine or have an interest in this area?

We are a national leader in supporting professional development and education.

Member benefits:

- Regional groups in the UK and internationally that provide local networking opportunities, workplace visits and clinical lectures
- Our acclaimed *Occupational Medicine* journal
- The SOM Learning Hub – with reports on the value of OH, resources and guidance leaflets
- Occupational health nurse indemnity insurance and free nurse appraisal online toolkit
- A monthly online newsletter including events, job advertisements and important policy and practice updates
- Free legal advice
- Access to our quality assured appraisal scheme to support revalidation
- Online / distance learning through our CPD accredited webinar package
- Discounted tickets to our Annual Conference
- Peer to peer support
- Access to our SOM Members website, with its resources and learning zone
- Preferential rates on doctor indemnity insurance
- Special interest groups e.g. on MSK, HAVS, Skin, and Mental Health, plus a CESR support group
- Free SOM App – renew membership, book events, view past webinars and access OH news and blogs
- 40% discount on the *Art and Occupation* book

For further information, please contact membership@som.org.uk

www.som.org.uk/membership-information

𝕏 @SOMNews